CHRONIC MYELOID LEUKEMIA

A Handbook for Oncologists and Hematologists

Tariq I. Mughal, MD, FRCP, FACP
*Clinical Professor of Medicine,
Tufts Medical Center, Boston, USA;
Consultant Physician in Hematology
and Medical Oncology, Denver, USA
and London, UK*

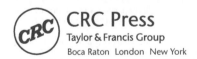

CRC Press
Taylor & Francis Group
Boca Raton London New York

CRC Press is an imprint of the
Taylor & Francis Group, an **informa** business

CRC Press
Taylor & Francis Group
6000 Broken Sound Parkway NW, Suite 300
Boca Raton, FL 33487-2742

© 2013 by Taylor & Francis Group, LLC
CRC Press is an imprint of Taylor & Francis Group, an Informa business

No claim to original U.S. Government works

Printed on acid-free paper
Version Date: 20130308

International Standard Book Number-13: 978-1-84214-577-7 (Paperback)

Visit the Taylor & Francis Web site at
http://www.taylorandfrancis.com

and the CRC Press Web site at
http://www.crcpress.com

"Clinicians of a certain age will remember the days when patients with CML filled our bone marrow transplant centers and often died of progressive disease despite our best efforts. In the past decade, we have been privileged to witness and contribute to a revolution in the basic, translational, and clinical science of CML that has dramatically improved the prognosis for these patients and served as a paradigm for the current effort in targeted therapy of cancer. In this volume, Dr. Tariq Mughal chronicles the history of this field and provides succinct and reasoned analyses of the current treatment approaches and controversies in CML. Both the general practitioner and the specialist will find much of value herein."

Richard Van Etten, MD, PhD, Professor of Medicine, Chief, Division of Hematology/Oncology, Tufts Medical Center, Boston, Massachusetts, USA

"In this handbook, Professor Mughal has written a comprehensive yet highly readable text on CML. It includes historical reference, clinical pearls, molecular biology, and common sense in a clear, organized manner. You will even find inclusion of the humanities (references to history and literature!) and humor, all of which so sadly missing from most scholarly works. One of the sad unintended consequences of the Internet Age is the assumption that everything can be found on the Web. Well, good luck in assembling the breadth of information contained in this handbook. Reader, do not waste your time jumping from one Internet link to another, trying to distinguish fact from fiction, and organizing the information into digestible content. Find a nice chair, a good light, and enjoy—Dr. Mughal has done the work for you. All you need to do is read, learn, and transmit your new knowledge to your patients' care."

Jerry Radich, MD, Professor of Medicine, Fred Hutchinson, Cancer Research Center, Seattle, Washington, USA

"This is a fantastic book written by a single author."

Professor Rüdiger Hehlmann, Medizinische Fakultät Mannheim der Universität Heidelberg, Heidelberg, Germany

"Professor Mughal is a world renowned leader in the field of molecular pathogenesis and therapy of chronic myeloid leukemia (CML). This illustrative handbook provides essential insights into the paradigmatic role of CML research in guiding the inception and maintenance of molecularly targeted therapy. The robust genetic dissection of CML blastic transformation and therapeutic resistance has informed the development of diagnostic and prognostic tools as well as therapeutic strategies that reach far beyond CML to a broad array of recalcitrant malignancies. Enjoy!"

Catriona Jamieson, MD, PhD, Associate Professor of Medicine, Division of Hematology-Oncology, Director for Stem Cell Research, Moores UCSD Cancer Center, La Jolla, California, USA

"Imatinib in chronic myeloid leukemia (CML) provided the first example of BCR-ABL–targeted therapy and based on this, there is currently considerable interest in the development of new JAK2 inhibitor drugs in classic Ph-negative MPN. I believe that lessons from CML pathophysiology and therapy provide benefits for MPN and many other cancers. Tariq's solo effort is a remarkable effort which summarizes the current state of affairs. I recommend it very highly."

Professor Tiziano Barbui, Bergamo, Italy

For
Sakina I. Mughal
(Ummi)

Acknowledgments

I thank my patients and my parents for having faith in me. I thank John Goldman, Beppe Saglio, Rick Van Etten, Jerry Radich, Catriona Jamieson, Rüdiger Hehlmann, Tiziano Barbui, and Ayalew Tefferi for reading the draft versions of the book, their comments, and their friendship. My gratitude, too, goes to Hérve Hoppenot, Bill Robinson, Nicholas Sarlis, Sergio Giralt, Hagop Kantarjian, Raj Chopra and many others for their support. I thank Robert Peden, Claire Bonnett and the CRC publishing team for their help and patience; Alpa and Sabena for their love.

Contents

Preface

The past three decades have witnessed chronic myeloid leukemia (CML), a clonal disease that results from an acquired genetic change in a single pluripotential hemopoietic stem cell, to have been served remarkably well by advancements in cellular and molecular biology. The speed at which these findings were translated to one of the great cancer medicine success stories of the past three decades is remarkable. Although CML is a rare disease, the lessons learned have led to a major paradigm shift in cancer medicine in general. For CML patients, the introduction of the tyrosine kinase inhibitor, imatinib mesylate, in 1998 was an important therapeutic milestone with most patients achieving a complete cytogenetic response and prolongation of survival compared with the previous therapies, other than stem cell transplantation. With the more recent regulatory approval in USA and many other countries of the second generation of tyrosine kinase inhibitors, dasatinib and nilotinib for first-line therapy of CML in chronic phase, and other candidate drugs in clinical trials, the pace at which the treatment algorithm for patients with CML is changing is unprecedented. There is however some uncertainty with regard to how best to assess efficacy of these and other potential next-generation drugs, such as ponatinib, in particular with regards to the most appropriate surrogate markers for overall survival. Currently the first-line studies of nilotinib use molecular markers and dasatinib use cytogenetic responses. There are also important differences in the precise definitions of common endpoints, such as event-free survival, progression-free survival and others.

In this inaugural edition of the CML handbook, I aim to provide important preclinical and clinical aspects of CML, for hematologists, oncologists and other health professionals interested in the disease. The opinions expressed are mine and I apologize for any errors or omissions.

TIM
Boston
January 2013

Foreword by John Goldman

The gradual unraveling of the mysteries of chronic myeloid leukemia is undoubtedly one of the greatest success stories of medicine over the last 50 years. The discovery of the cytogenetic events in the 1970s, following the landmark discovery of the Philadelphia chromosome in 1960, and the molecular events in the 1980s led to the seminal work by Brian Druker and his colleagues in the 1990s. These investigators found that a small molecule, now known as imatinib, could selectively block the enzymatic action of the ABL component of the BCR–ABL oncoprotein, which in turn led to the death of leukemia cells while leaving intact the residual nonleukemic hematopoietic cells in the marrow. Now, around 65% of patients who start imatinib while their disease is still in the chronic phase fare extremely well. At the eight-year mark, these patients show every sign of maintaining their good response for many more years and perhaps of achieving a life expectancy no different from a person of similar age without leukemia. This is a truly remarkable achievement for a disease which 20 years ago had a median life expectation of approximately five years from diagnosis.

Tariq Mughal's handbook on CML is both timely and authoritative, and this is understandable given his long-standing interest and training on the subject, which developed during the 1980s at the Hammersmith Hospital, London. The special merit of this handbook is that it combines breadth with depth. In one succinct volume you have the clinical history of CML, its natural history, its cytogenetic basis, and its molecular foundation (so far as this is known). In addition it details CML's avenues for clinical diagnosis in 2013, the current systems for clinical staging, and modern approaches to therapy which is linked with molecular monitoring for responding patients.

The therapeutic algorithms in this handbook provide a useful starting point for those not completely familiar with optimal management of CML in the current context. As the handbook is written by one author, the story runs in a logical order and avoids duplication.

Controversial issues are very well addressed; for example, the author correctly alludes to the uncertainty which exists in pediatric hematology, such as whether a child with newly diagnosed CML who does have a matched sibling should proceed straight to allografting or should receive an initial trial of imatinib and perhaps no allograft at all? Another controversy which is astutely addressed is whether the role of the new tyrosine kinase inhibitors and the concepts to accord a potential "cure."

Arguably the story of CML could well be a model for understanding and eventually treating other hematologic malignancies. There are few malignancies where the apparent initiating molecular events are as well characterized as they are in CML. Reading this comprehensive handbook will inform readers of past events, help them to decide how best to manage individual patients, and importantly, will provide inspiration to the notion that the problem of treating malignant diseases could indeed be solved within the next few decades.

John Goldman DM, FRCP, FRCPath
Emeritus Professor of Haematology
Imperial College London
London, UK
January 2013

Foreword by Giuseppe Saglio

It gives me great pleasure to write this foreword. I thought it would be fair to write a few lines about the author of this seminal handbook also. We may consider Tariq Mughal to be an important scientist, an experienced clinician, a clinical researcher and an international key opinion leader. The most fitting description of this and some of Tariq's other works, in my view is that he is an architect who enjoys building bridges. These are special and virtual bridges, but with the same function as the real ones—to connect people. This concise, yet thorough, handbook indeed provides a bridge between those who can be defined as "experts" on CML and those who want to further understand and to be updated on one of the most intriguing topics in cancer medicine in recent years.

CML is certainly an important type of leukemia from an epidemiological perspective. However, it may also be asserted that that its importance has further reach than that of a single disease. Indeed, CML provides a model to study and to dissect myeloid leukemias and possibly other hematological and nonhematological malignancies. We can also add that it is an "almost perfect model" as it allows to study at the same time, but clearly separated in different phases of the disease, the mechanisms leading to proliferation of the leukemic clone, those responsible for the block of apoptosis and those leading to a block of differentiation. There is a common and initial motor of all these altered events, the BCR–ABL tyrsoine kinase activity, that on one side promotes the initial proliferation and survival of the clone and on the other progressively stimulates its transformation from a rather benign disease into a terrible clinical entity that we have to slaughter well in advance to save the patients. The introduction and the success of imatinib into clinical practice a decade ago has further added to the intellectual appeal of CML. On one hand it has introduced the wheedling idea that our intelligence and knowledge can finally defeat cancer and on the other hand it has further added to the completeness of the model, as we can finally "switch off" (or at least slow down) the motor of the cancer and "see what happens." This is usually something we are only able to do *in vitro* or *ex vivo*. This further underlines the importance of Tariq's "bridge-building" skills in this volume: It not only links the experts and the less specialized, but also the basic researchers and the clinicians. The latter of these linkages can provide vital information, because if clinical inputs are observed with care and intelligence much can be revealed with regard to the biology of the disease.

This handbook is to be lauded for its capacity to augment the knowledge of specialists and nonspecialists comprehensively, while providing visionary scope for future developments in CML and beyond.

Professor Giuseppe Saglio, MD
Department of Clinical
and Biological Sciences
University of Turin, Turin, Italy
January 2013

1 An introduction to chronic myeloid leukemia

During the past three decades patients with hematological malignancies, particularly chronic myeloid leukemia (CML), have been served well by clinical and laboratory research and the unraveling of some of the molecular mechanisms that underlie malignant diseases has paved the way to defining potential specific targets for treatment. The success of such treatments, epitomizing the "bench-to-bedside" paradigm, has increased optimism for their broader application in cancer medicine.

CML, sometimes referred to as chronic myelogenous leukemia or chronic granulocytic leukemia, is a clonal *BCR–ABL1*-positive myeloid leukemia. In the World Health Organization's updated classification of myeloid malignancies (2008), CML is one of the myeloproliferative neoplasms (MPN). MPN comprises several rather heterogeneous, but well-characterized hematological malignancies: CML, polycythemia vera (PV), essential thrombocythemia (ET), primary myelofibrosis (PMF), mastocytosis, chronic eosinophilic leukemia not otherwise specified, chronic neutrophilic leukemia, and MPN, unclassifiable. CML, PV, ET, and PMF collectively are often referred to as "classic" MPN because they were included in the original description of "myeloproliferative disorders" by William Dameshek in 1951.

CML is thought to result from an acquired genetic change in a pluripotential hematopoietic stem cell. In the majority of patients, this genetic change results in a balanced translocation between chromosomes 9 and 22, t(9; 22) (q34; q11); the resulting 22q- is known as the Philadelphia (Ph) chromosome (Fig. 1.1).

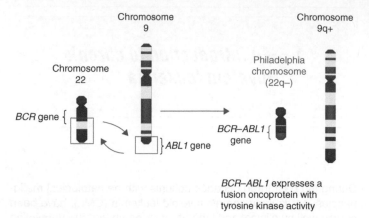

Figure 1.1
A schematic representation of the "origin" of the Philadelphia (Ph) chromosome.

All the leukemic progeny of the CML stem cell have this consistent cytogenetic abnormality, the Ph chromosome. The balanced translocation results in a *BCR–ABL1* fusion gene, which is associated with an oncoprotein, P210. In the early 1990s, following the demonstration that introducing the *BCR–ABL1* gene into murine stem cells in experimental animals caused a disease simulating human CML, this fusion gene and its related oncoprotein, which has an enhanced tyrosine kinase activity, have generally been accepted as the principal pathogenetic event leading to the chronic phase (CP) of CML.

CML is typically, at least historically, a biphasic or, sometimes a triphasic disease that often presents in the initial CP and then evolves spontaneously into an advanced phase, termed blast crisis (BC); this can sometimes occur via an accelerated phase, culminating into BC. BCR–ABL1 is now generally accepted to also be a principal cause for BC of CML. BCR–ABL1 has been shown to cause DNA damages and impairment of DNA repair, which leads to an accumulation of mutations, deletions, and chromosomal aberrations in the course of CML (Table 1.1). BCR–ABL1 independence is acquired by genetic instability.

In the mid-1990s, the discovery that this excessive kinase activity could be inhibited in a highly specific manner was a major landmark

Table 1.1
BCR–ABL1-Independent and TKI-Dependent Pathways to CML in BC

BCR–ABL1-independent
- Preexisting genomic instability
- Lyn kinase
- Microenvironment

TKI-dependent
- Clonal selection of BCR–ABL1 mutants
- TKI-induced genomic instability

Abbreviations: CML, chronic myeloid leukemia; TKI, tyrosine kinase inhibitor.

in the treatment of CML. Clinical studies using a small molecule tyrosine kinase inhibitor (TKI), imatinib mesylate (imatinib) (Glivec; also known as Gleevec; Novartis Pharma, Basel, Switzerland, previously known as CIBA-Geigy, Basel, Switzerland), as a single-agent treatment for patients with CML began in 1998 and showed that most patients achieved hematological and eventually complete cytogenetic responses (CCyR). Remarkably, by May 2001, the drug was licensed for first-line therapy of CML patients. Imatinib reduces substantially the number of leukemia cells in a patient's body and by 2003 there appeared promises to prolong survival substantially in comparison with previous therapy.

The drug's unprecedented clinical success has since been confirmed. It clearly alters the natural history of CML and the associated overall prognosis. A decade since imatinib gained regulatory approval for frontline use in patients with CML in the CP, it is evident that a significant majority of patients, those who achieve a CCyR within two years of initiating treatment, can anticipate an overall survival (OS) that is similar to that of the general population. Remarkably the estimated eight-year OS with imatinib is now considered to be about 85%, rising to about 93% if one considers only CML-related deaths (Fig. 1.2).

Responses are also seen in patients in the advanced phases of the disease, although these are generally not so impressive and not long-lasting in the majority. The MD Anderson Cancer Center

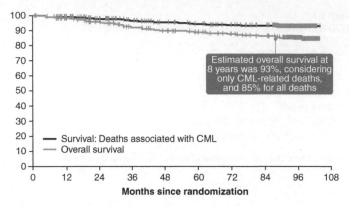

Figure 1.2
Leukemia-free survival based on the International Randomized trial of Interferon-α and cytarabine versus STI571 (an intention to treat analysis). Source: *Courtesy of Professor Michael Deininger, presented at ASH 2009.*

(MDACC) CML group published the survival data in January 2012 from 1569 patients, including 1148 patients in CP, and confirmed improvements in OS since 2001. Similar observations have been reported recently by a large Swedish study of 3173 patients diagnosed with CML treated over five decades and the German CML Study Group (see Figure 4.1b).

The responses are largely seen in patients in CP, but some are seen in the advanced phases also. These responses in patients who are in the advanced phases of CML are, however, interesting because whereas during the CP of the disease, the Ph chromosome is the sole cytogenetic abnormality present (supporting the notion of CML being a "one hit" disease caused by a single molecular abnormality), additional cytogenetic abnormalities ("second hits") are acquired as the disease progresses to the advanced phases. Thus responses in patients in BC serve as "proof of concept" that targeting a single initiating molecular abnormality can induce a response, at least transiently, in a cancer with multiple genetic abnormalities. Since most established cancers are thought to result from a series of genetic mutations, it is encouraging to note that responses akin to those seen in patients in blast phase of CML may occur if the initiating lesion alone can be targeted.

The majority of CML patients who respond well to imatinib still retain very small numbers of leukemia cells in their body. If imatinib were truly to "cure" CML, it would presumably have to eradicate leukemia cells, but laboratory studies suggest that a small subset of leukemia cells (some of which may be "quiescent" or transcriptionally silent stem cells) are insensitive to imatinib, even at doses up to 10 times the standard therapeutic dose. Thus patients who have responded extremely well to imatinib almost invariably "relapse" with increasing numbers of *BCR–ABL1* transcripts if for any reason imatinib treatment is interrupted, which suggests that even small numbers of surviving leukemia cells are capable of re-establishing the disease. This survival of leukemia "stem" cells able to acquire further mutations may also explain why some patients relapse directly in the advanced phases of CML from a complete cytogenetic response state.

About 30% of patients in CP and almost all of those in BC become resistant to the inhibitory effects of imatinib. Efforts have therefore focused largely, although not exclusively, on innovative methods to re-establish ABL1 tyrosine kinase inhibition. Some of these efforts led to the development of alternative inhibitors of ABL1 kinase activity, referred to as the second- or next-generation TKIs, which have now met a qualified success. These drugs include dual kinases inhibitors, such as dasatinib (Spyrcel; previously known as BMS-354825; Bristol–Myers Squibb, New York, New York, USA) and bosutinib (previously known as SKI-606; Pfizer, New York, New York, USA), which differ from imatinib in targeting multiple other kinases, such as SRC, in addition to the ABL1 kinase, and drugs such as nilotinib (Tasigna; previously known as AMN-107; Novartis, East Hanover, New Jersey, USA), an improved version of imatinib (Fig. 1.3).

More recently, the pan-BCR–ABL1 inhibitor, ponatinib (previously known as AP24534, Ariad Pharmaceuticals, Cambridge, Massachusetts, USA) also referred to as a third generation TKI, has been added to these agents (Table 1.2). Other drugs of interest include rebastinib (DCC-2036; Deciphera Pharmaceuticals, Lawrence, Kansas, USA), danusertib (PHA-739358; Nerviano Medical Sciences, Nerviano, Italy), and omacetaxine mepesuccinate (Omapro; previously known as homoharringtonine; Teva-Cephalon Oncology, Frazer, Pennsylvania, USA), all of which are now either in preclinical or clinical trials.

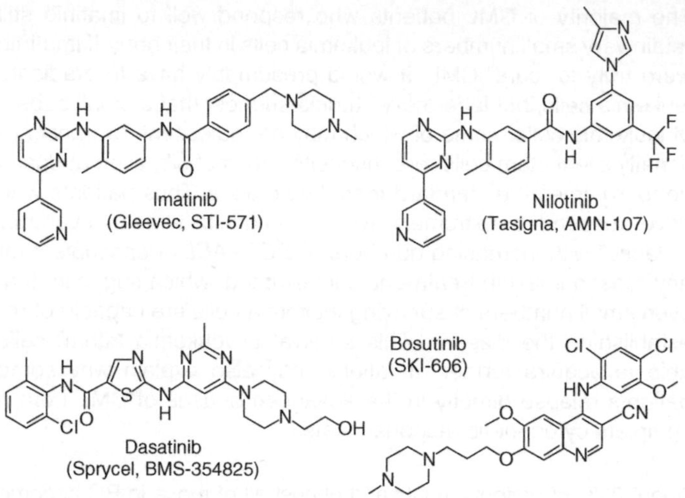

Figure 1.3
BCR–ABL1 *inhibitors.*

Table 1.2
Other New Emerging and Investigational Drugs for CML

T315I-active inhibitors
• Ponatinib, Rebastinib (DCC-2036), Danusertib (PHA-739358)
Nonkinase inhibitors
• Omacetaxine mepesuccinate, arsenic trioxide

Abbreviation: CML, chronic myeloid leukemia.

These drugs were initially tested in patients with CML who were either refractory or intolerant to imatinib, and following the confirmation of significant clinical efficacy and acceptable toxicity profile, all three drugs (dasatinib, nilotinib, and bosutinib, in that order) entered clinical trials assessing the drugs' potential first-line treatment role. Remarkably, current results from randomized phase III studies, suggest that these drugs, in particular dasatinib and nilotinib, may be more effective than imatinib. Both of these drugs received accelerated regulatory approval for first-line use in patients with CML in CP by the US Food and Drug Administration (FDA) and Switzerland in late 2010 and thereafter by the European

Medicines Agency (EMEA); in December 2011, nilotinib, but not dasatinib, was also approved by the National Institute for Health and Clinical Excellence (NICE) in the UK.

Randomized studies of nilotinib and dasatinib, compared with imatinib, have demonstrated significantly higher rates of CCyR and of major molecular response (MMR) at the landmark 12 months of follow-up, resulting in the regulatory approval. The studies also show a reduction in the risk of transformation to advanced phases of the disease, and in general better tolerance (so far). There are important differences between the two drugs, not simply in the trial design and endpoints, but also in the frequency and rate of responses, progression-free survival, and side effects. Bosutinib failed to meet its primary endpoint at 12 months in the randomized phase III trial and further studies are ongoing. The 12 months CCyR responses were not significantly different between the bosutinib and imatinib arms (70% vs. 68%, respectively); interestingly, the 12 months MMR were significantly different (39% vs. 26%, respectively). Bosutinib, however, was licensed in September 2012 for patients with CML who have failed previous TKI therapy. The next candidate drug, ponatinib, has demonstrated efficacy and reasonable safety in the pivotal phase II trial (PACE) and the drug was licensed in December 2012 for patients with CML and Ph-positive acute lymphoblastic leukemia (ALL) who have failed prior TKI therapy or harbor a T315 mutation. Ponatinib's candidacy for first-line therapy is currently being tested in a phase III trial, compared to imatinib.

Importantly, however, only a small minority of patients achieve long-term complete molecular response (CMR) with imatinib, and the frequency of CMR with the second-generation TKIs remains to be seen. Moreover, *in vitro* studies suggest that none of the TKIs eradicates quiescent CML stem cells, which may account for relapse in most, but not in all patients, once the drug is discontinued. It is therefore possible that none of the currently available TKIs will ultimately translate to a cure, as defined by the absence of all malignant cells. It is, of course, likely that an "operational" cure is achieved whereby most patients who achieve a CMR have very low levels of residual disease, which might not shorten the OS. In an attempt to achieve a conventional cure, many efforts are being directed to develop other treatments, such as immunotherapy and innovative combinations of TKIs and other drugs.

The remarkable success obtained with imatinib when used as first-line treatment of patients with CML in CP significantly changed the treatment algorithms that were in place a decade ago. The preferred treatment then was an allogeneic stem cell transplant (SCT) using an HLA-identical or a suitable matched unrelated donor, carried out as early as possible in the CP.

Such a treatment was able to accord long-term success to the majority of patients who were eligible for the procedure. Unfortunately, largely due to the lack of finding a suitable donor for most patients and the fact that the median age of patients with CML was around 63 years of age (when the risks associated with transplantation began to increase), most patients received interferon-α (IFN-α), which then became the preferred nontransplant treatment. IFN-α accorded complete hematological responses (CHR) to the majority of patients with CML in CP, but CCyR to only about 10–15%. The drug, however, was associated with significant side effects affecting the quality of life of most patients; the availability of the pegylated interferon formulation in the mid-1990s improved the drug's side effects considerably. It is of interest to note that in many of the patients who did achieve a CCyR on IFN-α therapy, the responses tended to spread over 10 years. It has now been suggested that the drug may target CML stem cells, a feat which none of the currently available TKIs seem to do. These observations provide some rationale for the notion of combining IFN-α with TKIs for first-line therapy.

There is now general agreement that most new patients should first receive treatment with a TKI. There are perhaps two exceptions to this general rule. First, some pediatricians feel that the results of allogeneic SCT in children are so comparatively good that it is reasonable to offer children with matched donors an allograft as initial treatment or after cytoreduction for a finite period with imatinib. Others feel that a child responding well to imatinib should be continued indefinitely on this agent. Thus for treating children there seems at present no general consensus. Second, a case can be made for transplanting as initial therapy patients for whom the cost of imatinib continued over many years would be totally prohibitive. For such patients a one-off procedure involving allografting might be a better option.

The question whether treatment to an adult should start with standard dose imatinib or to embark on treatment with a second-generation TKI cannot be resolved at present. We have more than 10 years experience with imatinib and over half of all the patients appear to be doing remarkably well. We have only very limited experience with the use of second-generation TKIs as initial therapy but preliminary results, with at least a 24 months follow-up, suggest that both nilotinib and dasatinib are superior to imatinib in terms of achieving molecular and cytogenetic responses and it is generally accepted that both drugs could replace imatinib as the preferred treatment for newly diagnosed patients with CML in CP. A further follow-up should help establish firmly the candidacy of either second-generation TKIs to be used as frontline therapy. Parenthetically, there is as yet no difference in survival between any of the arms in the nilotinib or dasatinib randomized trials. The decision-making process is facilitated by adopting validated guidelines.

Finally it is clear that as we understand the cellular and molecular biology of CML better and improve the prognosis for the vast majority of patients, we identify new questions and issues. Some of these include the challenge of identifying the important early endpoints of therapy with TKI that help predict long-term prognosis, optimizing monitoring response to therapy (cytogenetics, fluorescent in-situ hybridization, molecular studies, mutational analysis), and identification of the long-term endpoints important for therapy-related decisions and others.

Most of these successes, challenges, and strategies are addressed in this handbook.

2 A historical perspective of chronic myeloid leukemia

INTRODUCTION

The story of what we now know as chronic myeloid leukemia (CML) began in the early 19th century as a result of astute clinical observations. Thereafter, with the dawn of the era of medical microscopy and the use of aniline-based dyes to stain human tissues, leukemias were recognized as a distinct nosological entity. Many of the initial efforts focused on therapy and led to the introduction of arsenicals in the later part of the 19th century for symptomatic relief. This was largely supplanted by the introduction of ionizing radiation at the beginning of the 20th century and later by the alkylating agent, busulfan. Major progress in both the therapy and, indeed, the understanding of the disease did not occur until 1960 when advancements in the technology of cytogenetics led to the discovery of a consistent chromosomal abnormality in bone marrow cells of patients with CML. This was later termed the "Philadelphia" or (Ph^1) chromosome to acknowledge the city where the discovery took place. The era of molecular biology unfolded in the early 1980s, and led to the molecular unraveling of the "pathogenetic" or apparent "initiating" event for the chronic phase (CP) of CML. This, in turn, paved the way to the successful introduction of the original ABL kinase inhibitor, imatinib, as the preferred initial treatment of newly diagnosed patients in CP. The chronology of evolution of therapy is summarized in Figure 2.1.

THE 16TH TO 18TH CENTURIES

Claims of priority can almost always be challenged but it is generally agreed that microscopy was first introduced by Robert Hooke in England in 1665 and by Anton van Leeuwenhoek in the

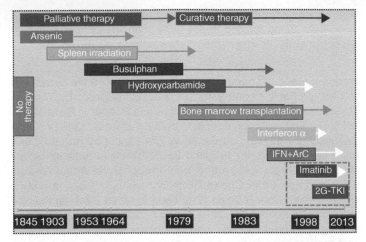

Figure 2.1
Historical evolution of treatment for patients with chronic myeloid leukemia in chronic phase (1845–2012).

Netherlands in 1674. Many efforts were undertaken thereafter to study blood cells. Initial descriptions of red blood cells appear to have been made by Jan Swammerdam in 1668 and Leuwenhoek in the Netherlands in 1674, and of white blood cells by Joseph Lieutaud in France in 1749 and William Hewson in England around 1765. The description of platelets, however, did not occur until the 19th century, just ahead of the efforts led by Paul Ehrlich in Germany and in the use of chemical dyes for better morphological assessment of the various blood cells.

THE 19TH CENTURY

Although Alfred Velpeau in France is credited with the first detailed description of what must have been leukemia in 1827, the first plausible references to the entity now known as CML were probably made in 1845, almost simultaneously, by John Bennett in Edinburgh, and Rudolf Virchow in Berlin. Both patients were noted to have very large spleens and an unusual consistency of the blood, which Virchow described as "weisses blut" and for which Bennett proposed the term "leucocythaemia."

In 1868 Ernst Neumann in Germany introduced the concept of blood cells being formed in the bone marrow and the notion of "leucocythemia" arising in the marrow rather than the spleen.

From a therapeutic perspective, efforts to improve the symptoms of CML probably began with the use of arsenicals by Thomas Fowler, but its use is first documented by Lissauer in Germany in 1865. The first report of arsenic to treat a patient with the probable diagnosis of CML was published in *The Lancet* by Arthur Conan Doyle from Birmingham, England, in 1882; there is some ambiguity about the letter since the author's name appears as Arthur 'Cowan' Doyle and not Arthur Conan Doyle, but this is probably merely a printer's error! Conan Doyle is, of course, rather more famous for his stories of Sherlock Holmes. Blood transfusion was performed, but largely without success, and did not become a safe procedure until the discovery of the human blood groups by Landsteiner in 1935. Splenectomy was also used but often resulted in the death of the patient.

THE 20TH CENTURY

In 1926, Minot and colleagues described the clinical features of CML in a classical paper. The notion of trilineage hematopoietic proliferation was introduced by Vaughan and Harrison in 1939 when they described two cases of "leucoerythroblastic anemia and myelosclerosis" and suggested that the trilineage proliferation arose from a "common primitive reticulum cell." By now efforts were in place to recognize "myeloproliferative diseases" as a separate entity from "acute leukemias." In 1951, William Dameshek, who started the journal *Blood* in USA, grouped CML with polycythemia vera, essential thrombocythemia, and myelosclerosis, and called the diseases collectively "chronic myeloproliferative diseases" in a seminal *Blood* editorial.

In 1960 Peter Nowell and David Hungerford, in Philadelphia, described the presence of an abnormally small acrocentric chromosome, which resembled a Y chromosome, in two male patients with what was then called chronic granulocytic leukemia. They subsequently described the presence of this chromosomal abnormality in a further seven patients, including two females, with CML. They then speculated that the abnormal chromosomal abnormality was probably not constitutive and may well be causally associated to CML. This abnormality was heralded as the first consistent cytogenetic abnormality in a human malignancy and was named Philadelphia (Ph[1]) chromosome, after the city of its discovery. The superscript "1" was added on the premise that additional abnormalities originating from Nowell and Hungerford's work would be discovered in Philadelphia. This, of course, did not occur and the superscript had been dropped by 1990. The formal recognition that a human cancer might be caused by an acquired chromosomal aberration, of course, vindicated to some degree, the hypothesis postulated by Theodore Boveri, in Germany, in 1914 that cancer may be caused by acquired chromosomal abnormalities.

The next important observations which established that CML was a stem cell-derived clonal disease came from Phillip Fialkow and colleagues in 1967. They applied a genetic technique developed by Susumu Ohno, Ernest Beutler, and Mary Lyon, based on X chromosome mosaicism in females, and by demonstrating polymorphism in the X-linked glucose-6-phosphatase dehydrogenase locus, established the clonal nature of not only CML, but also polycythemia vera, essential thrombocythemia, and primary myelofibrosis.

In 1972, Janet Rowley, in Chicago, described the morphological aspects of the Ph chromosome in some detail and by applying the new Giemsa chromosome banding technique, was able to demonstrate, for the first time, how the balanced reciprocal translocation of genetic material between the long arms of chromosomes 9 and 22, t(9;22)(q34;q11) arose. She deserves credit for making an observation that strongly supported the notion that cytogenetic changes play an important role in leukemogenesis.

The molecular events underlying the genesis of the Ph chromosome began to unfold in 1982, when Nora Heisterkamp and colleagues in Rotterdam mapped to chromosome 9 the human homolog of the Abelson murine leukemia virus. In 1984, the same group, led by John Groffen, described that the ABL gene was translocated to the Ph chromosome in CML. Thereafter ensued a major effort to document that the *ABL* gene was at the breakpoint using Southern blotting with ABL probes to detect rearrangements. Further efforts led to the recognition of three separate breakpoint locations on the *BCR* gene on chromosome 22.

Thereafter a number of keynote parallel achievements enhanced the molecular understanding further, commencing with the 1984 demonstration by Konopka and Witte that BCR–ABL had increased tyrosine kinase activity relative to c-ABL. Subsequently, in 1985, Canaani, Collins, and colleagues described an 8.5-kb BCR–ABL (now renamed BCR–ABL1) transcript that expressed an oncoprotein. This was identified in the same year as p210[BCR–ABL] by Shvitelman, Stam, Ben-Neriah, and colleagues. In 1986, Daley, Witte, Baltimore, and colleagues described the assembly and sequencing of the complete BCR–ABL1 cDNA (b3a2 isoform) from K562 cells, and helped in providing the immunological proof that BCR–ABL fusion protein was the product of the 8.5 kb fusion transcript. The presence of the p190 BCR–ABL1 fusion protein in patients with Ph-positive ALL was described by Erickson, Chan, Hermans, and colleagues between 1985 and 1987.

In 1988, Kurzrock and colleagues described the presence of the Ph chromosome in all leukemic cells of the myeloid lineage, and in some B-cells and in a very small proportion of T-cells in CML patients. The transforming ability of these BCR–ABL1 fusion proteins was attributed to the enhanced tyrosine kinase activity by George Daley and David Baltimore, in Boston, in 1988. Then in 1990, Daley and Baltimore, now working with Richard Van Etten, demonstrated that the *BCR–ABL1* gene was the principal cause for the chronic phase of CML, when they successfully introduced the *BCR–ABL1* gene into murine stem cells and caused a disease simulating human CML in about 40% of the mice. Remarkably, within four weeks of this publication, Heisterkamp and colleagues demonstrated leukemia in 8 of 10 transgenic mice models in a similar experiment. These findings were later confirmed by work done by Elephanty and colleagues in Australia and Kelliher and colleagues in Boston and Los Angeles.

In 1996 a third breakpoint location was found by Pane and colleagues in Italy. Patients with the very rare Ph-positive chronic neutrophilic leukemia had a much larger BCR–ABL1 fusion protein, p230 *BCR–ABL1*. This was designated the microbreakpoint cluster region (μ-bcr) and results in e19a2 mRNA, which encodes a larger protein of 230 kDa (see Fig. 3.3). Table 2.1 summarizes the principal milestones in the study of CML.

The remarkable consistency of these breakpoint locations paved the way toward the development by Nicholas Cross and colleagues of polymerase chain reaction technology to amplify small quantities of residual disease that might be left behind after effective treatment. This technique is now considered to be an effective method for molecular monitoring of individual patients with CML and it is discussed in chapter 7.

In the first half of the 20th century, the treatment in general focused on an improvement in the quality of life by controlling the symptoms attributed to CML. In the early 1900s, radiotherapy to the spleen was introduced and became popular for control of splenic enlargement. Radioactive phosphorus was also used intermittently. Other treatment modalities used, with very limited success,

Table 2.1
Milestones in the Study of CML

1960	"Philadelphia" chromosome
1973	Philadelphia chromosome is t(9;22)
1982	ABL involved in t(9;22)
1984	Discovery of BCR on chromosome 22
1985	*BCR–ABL* chimeric mRNA
1985	p210[BCR-ABL] has enhanced tyrosine kinase activity
1987	p190[BCR-ABL] Ph-positive ALL
1990	p210[BCR-ABL] murine model simulating the human disease
1997	p230[BCR-ABL] in CNL

Abbreviations: CML, chronic myeloid leukemia; ALL, acute lymphoblastic leukemia; CNL, chronic neutrophillic leukemia.

included antileukocyte sera in 1932, benzene in 1935, urethane in 1950, and leukapheresis. Despite the significant mortality associated and controversial benefits achieved, the use of splenectomy continued well into the 20th century.

The first cytotoxic drug used in CML was an alkylating agent, busulfan, which was introduced largely by David Galton at the Royal Marden Hospital, London, in 1953. Galton then carried out a prospective comparison of busulfan and splenic radiotherapy, and showed a significant survival advantage for the cohort subjected to busulfan. Thereafter busulfan became the preferred treatment for all patients with CML. In 1961, Institorisz and colleagues introduced 1,6-dibromomannitol, as possible alternative for patients who did not respond or became refractory to busulfan.

Hydroxycarbamide (previously hydroxyurea), a ribonucleotide reductase inhibitor, was introduced into clinics in the early 1960s, largely as a result of efforts by Kennedy and colleagues, and it gradually became the treatment of choice for newly diagnosed patients in chronic phase. A randomized study confirmed the superiority of hydroxycarbamide over busulfan, but neither drug reduced the proportion of Ph-positive cells in the bone marrow or prolonged the overall survival significantly, since neither affects disease progression in CML.

The next major development in the treatment of CML was the introduction of the first biological therapy, interferon-α (IFN-α), by Moshe Talpaz and colleagues, in Houston, in 1983. This agent was able to reduce the proportion of Ph-positive cells in the bone marrow in some patients and a minority achieving complete cytogenetic response (CCyR). Subsequent prospective randomized studies comparing IFN-α with hydroxycarbamide and busulfan confirmed IFN-α's superiority. It prolonged life by one to two years and by early 1990, became the nontransplant treatment of choice for the majority of patients with CML. It is of note that the French prospective randomized study confirmed the slight advantage accorded by adding low-dose cytarabine to IFN-α; this combination was later used as the control arm of the landmark trial International Randomized trial of Interferon-α and cytarabine versus STI571 (IRIS) assessing imatinib mesylate as a potential first-line therapy for newly diagnosed patients with CML in chronic phase. Remarkably, some of the patients who achieved Ph negativity continued to remain Ph negative even years after the drug was discontinued. It is now known that in such cases, the drug might have been able to kill the leukemia stem cells (see chap. 7).

Although the original concept of bone marrow transplant was probably first advocated by Thomas Fraser in 1894, when he famously recommended that patients eat bone marrow "sandwiches" flavored with port wine (to improve taste), sporadic attempts at marrow transplantation were undertaken much earlier.

The modern era of bone marrow (now stem cell) transplant did not begin until research had gained a basic understanding of the histocompatibility system. Much of the pioneering work in stem cell transplantation was carried out in the early 1970s by Don Thomas (who was subsequently awarded a Nobel prize for his contributions) and colleagues in Seattle. The early results were, for the most part, disappointing, largely because patients were in the advanced phases of the disease and succumbed to either the disease or the complications of the transplant. However, in 1979 the Seattle group reported successful treatment of four patients with CML in chronic phase who were transplanted with marrow cells collected from their respective normal genetically identical twins. These efforts stimulated a number of investigators to initiate programs for transplanting CML patients in chronic phase using marrow cells from their respective HLA-identical sibling donors. The results were very encouraging and by early 1990s, the potential for allogeneic transplant to induce a cure for the majority of patients was recognized.

The precise mechanisms by which this cure is achieved, however, remains unclear, although it must, in large part, be owing to an immunological assault on residual leukemia cells in the patient, which has been designated the "graft-versus-leukemia" (GvL) effect. Hans Kolb gets considerable credit for the seminal observation that donor lymphocyte infusion could induce remission in CML patients relapsing after an allograft, which served as the proof of the GvL concept. Most, but not all, patients in whom *BCR–ABL1* transcripts are repeatedly undetectable at five years after their allogeneic stem cell transplant will remain negative for long periods thereafter and will probably never relapse.

Following the establishment of the central role of BCR–ABL1 in CML in 1990, efforts were made to develop a small molecule that could inhibit the deregulated tyrosine kinase activity of the BCR–ABL oncoprotein. The initial results of the ultimately successful program led by Brian Druker in Portland, Oregon, and Alex Matter in Basel, Switzerland, were published in 1996. They developed a small molecule, imatinib mesylate (imatinib), which selectively inhibited the ABL tyrosine kinase and thereby disrupted the oncogenic signals, which led to the development of CML. Imatinib entered phase I trials in 1998 and phase II trials in 1999. The results were considered convincing enough for regulatory agencies to approve the use of this oral drug for the treatment of CML considered to be resistant or refractory to IFN-α, in 2001, although the results of a phase III study were still awaited.

THE 21ST CENTURY

Imatinib has unequivocally established the principles that molecularly targeted treatment can work and the lessons learned have been successfully applied to changing the therapeutic approaches for several malignancies, including the three most common cancers in the western world, breast, lung, and colon. By 2005, it was also confirmed that imatinib resulted in a significant proportion of patients with CML in chronic phase achieving a CCyR and prolongation of survival compared with the historical therapies. However, the drug was not universally successful and an increasing proportion of patients were considered to have had a suboptimal response and even failure. Further efforts led to the introduction of the second-generation TKI, dasatinib, nilotinib, and bosutinib, initially for patients who had failed or where intolerant to imatinib and since 2010 both dasatinib and nilotinib, but not bosutinib, have been licensed for first-line therapy in CML patients. Both nilotinib and dasatinib have been shown to be more potent than imatinib and in randomized trials have demonstrated significantly higher rates of CCyR and of major molecular response at 12 months leading to the Food and Drug Administration (FDA) approval for first-line therapy for the treatment of newly diagnosed patients. We now have the 36 months follow-up for nilotinib and the 24 months follow-up for dasatinib, which is discussed in chapters 5 and 6.

3 Cytogenetics, molecular anatomy, and molecular biology of chronic myeloid leukemia

INTRODUCTION

The Philadelphia (Ph) chromosome is an acquired cytogenetic abnormality present in all leukemic cells of the myeloid lineage and in some B cells and T cells in patients with CML. It is formed as a result of a reciprocal translocation of genetic material of chromosomes 9 and 22 (Figs. 1.1 and 3.1). This balanced translocation results in a *BCR–ABL1* fusion gene on the Ph chromosome and also a "reciprocal" fusion gene, designated *ABL–BCR*, on the derivative 9q chromosome (der 9q+).

It is likely that the acquisition of the *BCR–ABL1* fusion gene by a hematopoietic stem cell and the ensuing expansion of the Ph-positive clone set the scene for acquisition and expansion of one or more Ph-positive subclones that are genetically more aggressive than the original Ph-positive population. The propensity of the Ph-positive clone to acquire such additional genetic changes is an example of "genomic instability," but the molecular mechanisms underlying this instability are poorly defined. Such new events may occur in the *BCR–ABL1* fusion gene or indeed in other genes in the Ph-positive population of cells.

The Ph-positive cell is prone to acquire additional chromosomal changes, presumably as a result of acquired "genetic instability," and this presumably underlies the progression to advanced phases of the disease. There is no consistent pattern of molecular abnormalities in patients whose disease has progressed from chronic phase. In this chapter some of the topical aspects of the

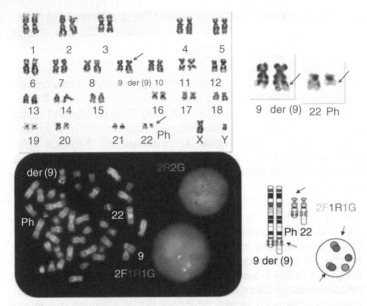

Figure 3.1
(i) Full and partial G banding of a Philadelphia (Ph) chromosome (+) cell (top) and (ii) BCR–ABL1 positive metaphase and interphase cell with florescent in situ hybridization (FISH) signals (2F1R1G) from D-FISH BCR–ABL1 probe (Vysis) along with a normal interphase nucleus (2R2G) for comparison on the left and a cartoon explaining the D-FISH pattern on the right (bottom half). Source: Courtesy of Dr Ellie Nacheva. A color version of this figure can be found in Plate I between pages 46 and 47.

cytogenetics, molecular anatomy, and molecular biology of chronic myeloid leukemia are reviewed.

CYTOGENETICS AND MOLECULAR ANATOMY

The Ph chromosome is an acquired cytogenetic abnormality that characterizes all leukemic cells in CML. It is formed as a result of a reciprocal translocation of chromosomal material between the long arms of chromosome 22 and chromosome 9, t(9; 22) (q34; q11). This balanced translocation results in a *BCR–ABL1* fusion gene on the Ph chromosome (see below) and also a "reciprocal" fusion gene, designated *ABL–BCR*, on the derivative 9q chromosome. Such translocations involving just two chromosomes are described as "simple," whereas about 10% of patients have "complex" translocations involving chromosomes 9, 22, and one or sometimes two other chromosomes.

In CML patients, the Ph chromosome is present in all myeloid cell lineages, in some B cells and in a very small proportion of T cells. It is found in no other cells of the body. This distribution is not altered by traditional treatment with busulphan or hydroxy-carbamide (previously known as hydroxyurea). Although valuable since the 1960s as a marker of the leukemic cell, its true pathogenetic significance remained uncertain until the identification of the *BCR–ABL1* chimeric gene on the Ph chromosome in the 1980s. About 15% of patients have small deletions of chromosomal material on der9q+, which usually include the reciprocal *ABL1–BCR* gene. Such deletions are thought to occur contemporaneously with the formation of the *BCR–ABL1* gene on the Ph chromosome and denoted a relatively poor overall prognosis in the pre–imatinib era; however, patients with der9q+ deletions respond as well to imatinib, and possibly to the second-generation tyrosine kinase inhibitors (TKIs; although this is not confirmed yet) as those lacking such deletions. A small proportion of patients with clinically classical CML lacks the Ph chromosome; however, most of these also have a typical *BCR–ABL1* gene expressed as a p210 oncoprotein (see below) and most have more complex cytogenetic abnormalities that probably mask the original t(9; 22).

Some, but not all, patients acquire additional clonal cytogenetic abnormalities during the course of the chronic phase. There was suspicion that some such changes might be caused in part by administration of alkylating agents, but they can undoubtedly occur spontaneously. The observation of nonrandom changes, typically 8, Ph, iso-17q, or 19, sometimes means that such new clones will expand and that blast crisis (BC), sometimes referred to as blastic transformation or blastic phase, will manifest itself within weeks or months, but these new clones (other than iso-17q) can remain clinically unimportant for many years. In overt BC, 80% of patients have clonal cytogenetic changes in addition to the Ph translocation.

It is generally believed that some CML stem cells, at a cytokinetic level, are in a quiescent or dormant (G_0) phase. These quiescent CML cells appear to be able to exchange between a quiescent and a cycling status, allowing them to proliferate under certain circumstances. This perhaps provides some rationale for *aficionados* of autografting to pursue this clinical research approach for patients with CML, almost 37 years since investigators from Seattle reported their initial experience! There is also evidence that some Ph-positive cells are quiescent and cannot be eradicated by cycle-dependent cytotoxic drugs, even at high doses, or indeed by any of the currently available TKIs (imatinib, dasatinib, nilotinib, or bosutinib).

MOLECULAR BIOLOGY

It was shown in the early 1980s that the *ABL1* proto-oncogene, which encodes a nonreceptor tyrosine kinase, was located normally on chromosome 9 but was translocated to chromosome 22 in CML patients. In 1984 the precise positions of the genomic breakpoint on chromosome 22 in different CML patients were found to be "clustered" in a relatively small 5.8-kb region to which the name "breakpoint cluster region" (BCR) was given. Later, it became clear that this region formed the central part of a relatively large gene now known as the *BCR* gene, whose normal function is not well defined, and the breakpoint region was renamed "*major* breakpoint cluster region" (M-BCR). In contrast, the position of the genomic breakpoint in the *ABL* gene (now often referred to as the *ABL1* gene to distinguish it from the ABL-related gene, *ARG* or *ABL2*) is very variable, but it always occurs upstream of the second (common) exon (a2). Thus, the Ph translocation results in juxtaposition of 5'-sequences from the *BCR* gene with 3'-ABL1 sequences derived from chromosome 9 (Fig. 3.2). It produces a chimeric gene, designated *BCR–ABL*, or better *BCR–ABL1*, which is transcribed as an 8.5-kb mRNA and encodes a protein with a molecular mass of 210 kDa. This p210[BCR–ABL1] oncoprotein has far greater tyrosine kinase activity than the normal *ABL1* gene product.

In CML, there are two variants of the *BCR–ABL1* transcript, depending on whether the break in M-BCR occurs in the intron

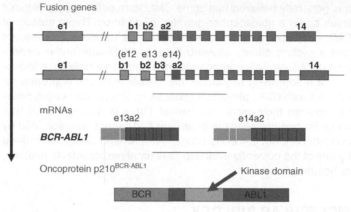

Figure 3.2
A schematic representation of the molecular anatomy of the Philadelphia (Ph) chromosome. A color version of this figure can be found in Plate I *between pages 46 and 47.*

between exons e13 and e14, or in the intron between exons e14 and e15. A break in the former intron yields an e13a2 mRNA junction and a break in the latter intron yields an e14a2 junction. (It should be noted that exon e13 was previously termed exon b2 and exon e14 was previously b3; thus the two RNA junctions were previously known as b2a2 and b3a2, respectively.) Most patients have transcripts with features of either e13a2 or e14a2, but occasional patients have both transcripts present in their leukemia cells. The precise type of *BCR–ABL1* transcript has no prognostic significance for CML patients. Moreover, the reciprocal *ABL–BCR1* gene on der9q⁺ is expressed in about 70% of patients, but its expression or lack of expression does not have prognostic significance.

A minority of patients with Ph-positive acute lymphoblastic leukemia (ALL), more often adults than children, also have *BCR–ABL1* fusion genes in their leukemia cells. In about one-third of Ph-positive ALL patients, the molecular features of the *BCR–ABL1* gene are indistinguishable from those of CML; in the remaining two-thirds the genomic breakpoint occurs in the first intron of the *BCR* gene (a zone designated M-BCR) and the *BCR–ABL1* gene results from fusion of the first exon (designated e1) of the *BCR*

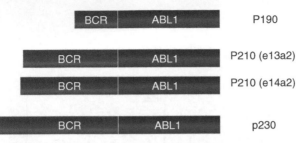

Figure 3.3
The various Ph-positive associated oncoproteins in human leukemias.

gene with the second exon (a2) of the *ABL1* gene. The mRNA is designated e1a2 and encodes a protein of 190 kDa (p190$^{BCR–ABL1}$) (sometimes reported in the literature as "P185"). Very rare patients with CML have a p190 protein instead of the usual p210. Equally rare is the finding of a Ph chromosome in association with chronic neutrophilic leukemia. Such patients may have an mRNA formed from an e19a2 fusion gene associated with a p230$^{BCR–ABL1}$ oncoprotein (Fig. 3.3).

The *BCR–ABL1* gene has been cloned and inserted into a retroviral vector that has been used to transfect murine hematopoietic stem cells; these transduced stem cells can generate a disease resembling human CML following transplantation into recipient mice. Thus, the *BCR–ABL1* gene is thought to play a (qualified) pivotal role in the genesis of chronic-phase CML. More recently there has been some speculation that at least in some patients, the initiating event might not be the *BCR–ABL1* gene. The mechanism by which the BCR–ABL1 oncoprotein alters stem cell kinetics remains ill-defined. It undoubtedly aberrantly autophosphorylates and also phosphorylates a wide range of intracellular proteins that would not normally be phosphorylated, including Crkl, MEK 1/2, RAC, and JNK. It may act by activating the RAS or STAT signal transduction pathways. Alternatively, it may activate the PI3 kinase/ AKT pathway involved in inhibiting apoptosis (Fig. 3.4). As an activated ABL1 opposes cellular apoptosis, the *BCR–ABL1* gene might act by impeding "programmed cell death" in target stem cells.

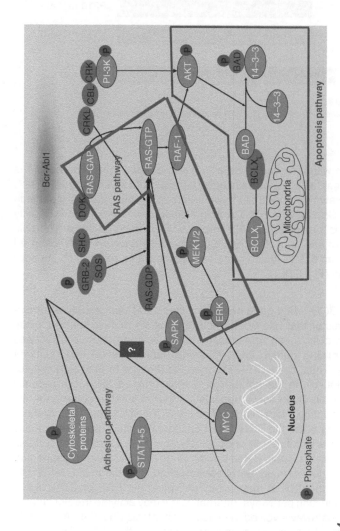

Figure 3.4
Signal transduction pathways which are potentially important in chronic myeloid leukemia in chronic phase.

The molecular basis of disease progression is still obscure, but it seems reasonable to infer that one or more probably a sequence of additional genetic events occurs in the Ph-positive clone. When the critical combination of additional events is achieved, clinically definable transformation ensues. At this stage, the leukemia cells usually harbor one or other of the additional cytogenetic changes referred to above. About 20% of patients with CML in myeloid transformation have point mutations or deletions in the coding sequence of the *p53* tumor suppressor gene, a gene implicated in progression of a variety of solid tumors, notably colonic carcinoma. The retinoblastoma (*RB*) gene is deleted in rare cases of CML in megakaryoblastic transformation, and changes in the *LYN*, *EVI-1*, and *MYC* genes are described. About half of the patients with lymphoid blast transformations have homozygous deletions in the p16 gene, whose normal function is to inhibit cyclin-dependent kinase 4. A recent work by Mullighan and colleagues demonstrate that the majority of Ph-positive B-ALL have loss-of-function mutations in genes regulating lymphoid development, including IKZF1, PAX5, and EBF; molecular changes underlying the nonrandom cytogenetic changes described above have not been identified.

As discussed in chapter 1, BCR–ABL1 has been shown to cause DNA damages and impairment of DNA repair, which leads to an accumulation of mutations, deletions, and chromosomal aberrations in the course of CML (Fig. 1.2 and Table 1.1). Other works of interest include that of Ito and colleagues observed that in a mouse model of CML, disease progression is regulated by the Musashi–Numb signaling axis. They found that the chronic phase was marked by high levels of Numb expression, whereas mice in BC phase had low levels of Numb expression. Collectively their data showed that the Musashi–Numb pathway can control the differentiation of CML cells. Perrotti and colleagues have demonstrated that several targets shared by BCR–ABL1 and PP2A are either essential for BCR–ABL1 leukemogenesis or are altered in CML in BC. They also observed the importance of restoration of PP2A activity in terms of regulation of survival, proliferation, self-renewal, and differentiation of CML, either by chemical PP2A activators (such as forskolin and FTY720) or by interfering with SET/PP2A interplay. By restoring normal PP2A activity, they were able to induce marked apoptosis of CML stem cells and suppress leukemogenesis regardless of sensitivity to imatinib or other TKIs.

PP2A-activating drugs, such as FTY720, also appear to eradicate CML stem cells, while sparing normal progenitors. It should be of interest to now assess this drug in trials for patients with CML in BC. Clearly these and other observations suggest future candidate targets which could be studied.

CONCLUSION

Although the observation that a small molecule such as imatinib could reverse the clinical and hematological features of CML constituted the final proof of the importance of the BCR–ABL1 oncoprotein to CML, there persisted some uncertainty about whether *BCR–ABL1* was the initiating lesion or only a secondary event. Indirect evidence, collated by Fialkow and colleagues in 1981, had suggested that there may be a preceding predisposition to genomic instability in a Ph-negative population. There are also rare case reports of families where multiple individuals have different myeloproliferative neoplasms, including polycythemia vera, essential thrombocythemia, and CML.

Clonal changes have now been seen in the Ph-negative populations in patients successfully treated for Ph-positive CML, especially 8, monosomy 7, and −Y. Occasional cases of patients with Ph-negative acute myeloid leukemia (AML) responding to imatinib have been reported. In 2007, Zaccaria and colleagues, in Rome, reported five CML patients who had multiple cytogenetic abnormalities coexisting in the Ph-positive cells of newly diagnosed CML patients; when the patients were treated with imatinib therapy the Ph chromosome was eliminated but the other abnormalities persisted. The authors speculated that the non-Ph abnormalities must have preceded the acquisition of the Ph chromosome. Furthermore, in 2007, Brazma and colleagues in London demonstrated that some patients with CML had predisposing molecular abnormalities identifiable by micro-array comparative genomic hybridization occurring within the Ph chromosome.

The BCR–ABL1 gene has, of course, been cloned and inserted into a retroviral vector that has been used to transfect murine hematopoietic stem cells, which can generate a disease resembling human CML in mice. Based on this it was generally accepted that the BCR–ABL1 gene must play a principal role in the genesis of the chronic phase of CML. For the moment, despite the slight uncertainty in some patients, and more importantly the irrefutable clinical benefit demonstrated by the various TKIs, most experts would acknowledge the unprecedented importance of the BCR–ABL1 gene, even in the rare patient in whom it might, or might not, be the initiating event for the chronic phase of the disease.

INTRODUCTION

The incidence of chronic myeloid leukemia (CML) worldwide, with the possible exception of India, appears to be fairly constant. It occurs in 1.0–1.5 per 100,000 of the adult population per annum. In the Western world it represents approximately 15% of all adult leukemias and <5% of all childhood leukemias but the percentage is higher in the East where chronic lymphocytic leukemia is rare. It is likely that in India the incidence is higher but the precise figures are not available at present. The median age of onset is around 55 years in the West, and, based on hospital registries, around 36 years in India. The disease appears to afflict more males than females.

Importantly as our efforts to treat patients with CML improve in the TKI era, the prevalence of the disease has increased: if the annual death rate is around 2%, this predicts 250,000 CML patients in USA by 2030 (Fig. 4.1A); similar estimates have been predicted for CML patients in Europe (Fig. 4.1B). Clearly if the annual death rate is now around 1%, as many CML specialists believe it to be so, then this predicts 500,000 CML patients by 2030!

Although in most cases there are no known predisposing factors, there is a marginally increased risk of developing CML following exposure to high doses of irradiation, as occurred in survivors of Hiroshima and Nagasaki atomic bombs in 1945. A small number of families with high incidence of the disease have been reported, and relapse of CML originating in donor cells following related donor allogeneic SCT has been recorded. Nevertheless, it is extremely difficult to incriminate any single etiological factor in individual patients with CML.

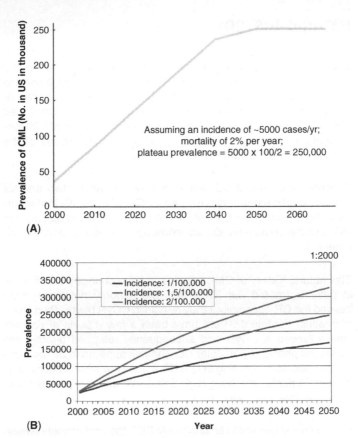

Figure 4.1
*Estimated prevalence of CML in (**A**) USA (courtesy of Professor Hagop Kantarjian);
(**B**) Europe from Hehlmann R. CML in the imatinib era. Best Pract Res Clin Hematol 2009;
22: 283–4.* Abbreviation: *CML, chronic myeloid leukemia. A color version of this figure can
be found in* Plate II *between pages 46 and 47.*

In May 2011 a Korean group published a report of a genome-wide
association study involving more than 3000 subjects (Korean and
European descent), which identified two candidate novel loci, 6q25.1
and 17p11.1, associated with susceptibility to CML. It was of interest
that the locus 6q25.1 was validated in both Korean and European
cohorts, whereas 17p11.1 only in the Korean cohort.

NATURAL HISTORY

CML is a remarkably heterogeneous disease. Historically, at least in the pre-TKI era, CML was a biphasic or triphasic disease that was usually diagnosed in the initial chronic phase, which used to last 5–10 years. Following this, the disease evolved spontaneously into an advanced phase, which could often be subdivided into an earlier accelerated phase and a later acute or BC. Parenthetically it should be noted that the precise definitions of the various phases have been much debated.

Patients with myeloid BC usually survived between two and six months; patients entering a lymphoid BC had a slightly better survival. About half of the patients in the CP transformed directly into BC and the remainder did so following a period of accelerated phase.

This natural history of CML appears to have changed significantly in patients treated with TKIs, with the majority not progressing beyond the CP, especially if they remain in CCyR beyond two years of imatinib treatment. There have been a few reports of patients who achieved a CCyR and subsequently relapsed directly into advanced phase, in particular BC. The risk appears to be the highest for patients presenting in late CP at the time when imatinib was started. Patients who have high Sokal-risk category disease also appear to fare less well.

For patients subjected to an allogeneic SCT, the vast majority remain in a complete cytogenetic response (CCyR) and complete molecular response (CMR) for 10 years or more. Some of these patients do become intermittently positive for *BCR–ABL1* transcripts, albeit at low levels, but the rare patient with a persisting high transcript level is at a high risk of relapse (Fig. 4.2). A very small minority appear to relapse directly into the advanced phases of the disease.

CLINICAL PRESENTATION

About one-third to one-half of the patients with CML are diagnosed in CP following a routine blood test, performed for unrelated reasons, and the remainder present with signs and symptoms

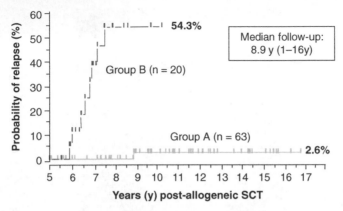

Figure 4.2
BCR–ABL1 transcripts following allogeneic SCT in patients treated at the Hammersmith Hospital, London, between 1981 and 1998. Abbreviation: *SCT, stem cell transplant.*
Source: *From Mughal TI, Yong A, Szydlo R, et al. RT-PCR studies in patients with chronic myeloid leukemia in remission 5 years after allogeneic stem cell transplant define risk of subsequent relapse. Br J Haematol 2001; 115: 569–74.*

related to anemia, platelet dysfunction, and splenomegaly (Fig. 4.3). Such symptoms may include lethargy, loss of energy, increased sweating, shortness of breath on exertion or weight loss, or hemorrhage from various sites. Spontaneous bruising or unexplained bleeding from gums, intestinal or urinary tract are relatively uncommon today. There may be pain or discomfort in the splenic area (Table 4.1). Very rarely, male patients may present with features of priapism. Most patients diagnosed in the advanced phases of CML tend to be symptomatic. Some patients with CML in BC can also present with skin involvement (leukemia cutis) (Fig. 4.4).

In about 95% of patients the diagnosis is typically made by the examination of a peripheral blood film (Fig. 4.5) and the demonstration of the Ph chromosome by conventional marrow cytogenetics; the remainder are diagnosed by the presence of a *BCR–ABL1* gene, although the use of fluorescence in situ hybridization (FISH) results in occasional false-negative results.

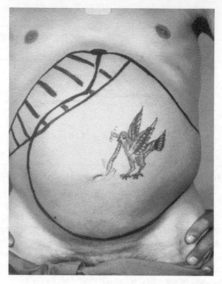

Figure 4.3
A patient with chronic myeloid leukemia presenting with a massive splenomegaly (and a wicked sense of humor).

Table 4.1
Clinical Features of Patients with Chronic Myeloid Leukemia in Chronic Phase

Clinical Feature	%
Fatigue	33.5
Bleeding	21.3
Weight loss	20.0
Abdominal discomfort (left upper quadrant)	18.6
Sweats	14.6
Bone pain	7.4
Splenomegaly	75.8
Hepatomegaly	2.2

Source: Savage D, Szydlo R, Goldman JM, et al. Clinical features at diagnosis of 430 patients with chronic myeloid leukemia seen at a referral centre over a 16-year period. Br J Haematol 1997; 96: 111–16.

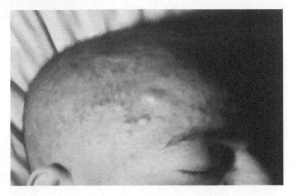

Figure 4.4
A patient with chronic myeloid leukemia in blast crisis and leukemia cutis. A color version of this figure can be found in Plate II *between pages 46 and 47.*

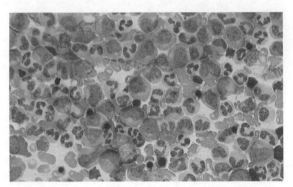

Figure 4.5
A photomicrograph of a peripheral blood film from a patient with chronic myeloid leukemia in chronic phase. A color version of this figure can be found in Plate III *between pages 46 and 47.*

Examination of the bone marrow by aspiration or trephine biopsy is not necessary to confirm the diagnosis of CML, but is usually carried out to assess the degree of marrow fibrosis, to perform cytogenetic analysis on marrow cells and to exclude incipient transformation. The marrow aspirate is often very hypercellular. Figure 4.6 depicts the typical features noted in a bone marrow biopsy (trephine) obtained from a patient with CML in myeloid blast crisis.

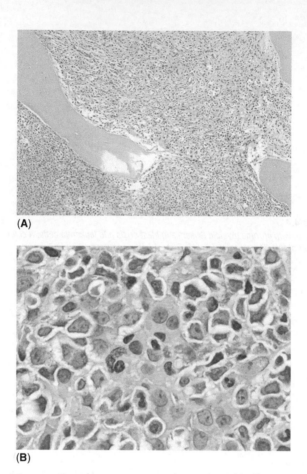

(A)

(B)

Figure 4.6
*Photomicrographs of bone marrow biopsy from a patient with chronic myeloid leukemia in myeloid blast crisis (**A**) low and (**B**) high magnification. A color version of this figure can be found in* Plate III *between pages 46 and 47.*

PROGNOSTIC AND PREDICTIVE FACTORS

In recognition of CML being heterogenous, efforts have been made to establish criteria definable at diagnosis that may help to predict survival for individual patients. Patients with CML in CP deemed as having a high probability of resistance or progression can be offered more aggressive therapy, for example, the use of initial second generation TKI, be enrolled in a clinical trial, or be considered for allogeneic SCT. In addition, patients at high risk could be monitored closely, with considerations for alternative or more aggressive therapy if strict optimal response criteria are not met.

At presentation, patients with CML are presumed to have acquired the original *BCR–ABL1* gene months or more probably years previously. The clinical and laboratory features that serve as surrogates of time from disease initiation are the spleen size and the white blood cell count (WBC). Although the rates at which the spleen grows and the WBC count increases vary among different patients, these parameters provide a gross estimate of disease burden. Prior to therapy, unopposed *BCR–ABL1* signaling promotes proliferation and genetic instability. Furthermore, it is possible that the longer the period of time elapsed between CML initiation and TKI therapy, the greater the likelihood of additional molecular mutations, which may lead to the more advanced phases of the disease.

Various clinical efforts have been made to establish criteria definable at diagnosis, both prognostic (disease-related) and predictive (treatment-related). Historically, the first useful method was that devised by Sokal and colleagues, in 1984, whereby patients were divided into various risk categories based on a mathematical formula that takes account of the patient's age, spleen size, blast cell count, and platelet count at diagnosis. Stratifying patients into good, intermediate, and poor risk categories may assist in the decision-making process regarding appropriate treatment options. This risk stratification method was based on 813 patients who were treated with conventional chemotherapy at six American and European centers and was initially referred to as "International index," but renamed "Sokal index," after Joseph Sokal's death in 1986. It is remarkable that although the Sokal score was developed for patients in CP being treated with hydroxyurea or busulfan, it also proved useful for predicting the outcome for patients treated with interferon, and now imatinib. It also appears to serve as a predictive factor for patients who are imatinib failures and are receiving second-generation TKIs, but this requires further confirmation. Regardless, the robustness of the Sokal score in varied clinical scenarios suggests that the score must allow for factors intrinsically related to CML cells and not simply factors present at diagnosis.

The European, or Hasford, scoring system was developed in 1997 based on 1573 patients who were treated with IFNα-based regimens at 12 European Institutes and patients where divided into three risk groups (Fig. 4.7). It was essentially an updated Sokal index, which incorporated the effects of increased basophil and eosinophil numbers. Importantly, both Sokal index and the Hasford score were validated by several groups following the introduction of imatinib. Both were shown to predict response but not survival. Table 4.2 depicts the calculation of relative risk (http://www.icsg.unibo.it/rrcal.asp) by Sokal and Hasford scores in patients with CML in CP.

It is also of interest that older age, a feature of both Sokal index and Hasford score, might not be of major prognostic relevance in

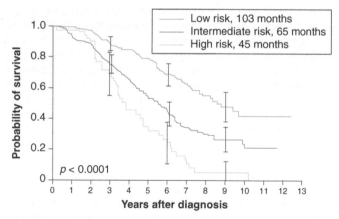

Figure 4.7
Probability of survival and median survival values for a population of chronic myeloid leukemia patients classified into low, intermediate, and high risk categories according to the Hasford (Euro) prognostic system (3). A color version of this figure can be found in Plate IV *between pages 46 and 47.*

imatinib-treated patients. Investigators from the MDACC (Houston) observed that among a cohort of 187 patients with CML in early CP, 87% of patients older than 60 years achieved a CCyR compared with 79% of patients younger than 60 years when treated with imatinib. This supports the notion that age *per se* does not influence the biology of the disease; rather the emergence of a potential comorbid condition in the older patient might increase the probability of treatment-related adverse effects.

Another possible prognostic factor, at least in the pre–imatinib era, was the presence or absence of deletions in the derivative (der) 9q+ chromosome. It is generally not considered to be significant in the imatinib era. This is also supported by the prognosis of patients with variant translocations, which frequently include der(9) deletions. In an analysis of 60 patients with CML and der(9) deletions (by FISH) who had been treated with imatinib, the Italian hematology group (GIMEMA) found no evidence of this conferring a poor

Table 4.2
Calculation of Relative Risk (http://www.icsg.unibo.it/rrcal.asp) by Sokal and Hasford Scores in Patients with CML in Chronic Phase

	International/ Sokal Score	European/ Hasford Score
Age (years)	0.116 (age − 43.4)	0.666 when age >50 years
Spleen size (cm)[a]	0.0345 × (spleen − 7.51)	0.042 × spleen
Platelet count (× 10^9/L)	0.188 × [(platelet/700)^2 − 0.563]	1.0956 when platelet count ≥ 1500
Blood blast cells (%)	0.0887 × (blast cells − 2.10)	0.0584 × blast cells
Blood basophils (%)	NA	0.20399 when basophils > 3%
Blood eosinophils (%)	NA	0.0413 × eosinophils
Relative risk	(Exponential of the total)	(Total × 1000)
Low	<0.8	≤780
Intermediate	0.8–1.2	781–1480
High	>1.2	>1480

[a]Maximum distance from costal margin.

prognosis. Other factors, such as the rate of shortening of telomerases, may help to define prognosis after a patient has started treatment.

More recently, the response to imatinib may predict for survival without progression to advanced phase. Historically, most of the studies conducted with imatinib, including the IRIS, as well as older therapies, in particular IFN-α, have suggested that the achievement of CCyR is associated with an improved survival. In contrast to this, there is some uncertainty as to whether achieving a MMR, defined by a *BCR–ABL1* ratio of <0.1% by International Scale, is associated with a better survival than achieving merely a CCyR. In the IRIS trial an earlier analysis confirmed that an MMR at 12 months was associated with an improved event-free survival (EFS), but not OS. A later analysis, however, failed to confirm this; rather it showed that achieving an MMR at 18 months, and not at 12 months, was now associated with a better EFS. Currently there appear to be diverse associations between MMR and survival at different milestones, compared with the impact of CCyR and survival. Consequently, many, although not all, experts concur that achievement of a CCyR on TKI should be the principal goal and the achievement of an MMR may confer additional benefit and is of secondary importance.

It is of considerable interest that several investigators are now exploring the potential to rely predominantly on *BCR–ABL1* transcript numbers at given time points to assess prognosis. The investigators identified transcript numbers at three months as the single most important prognostic factor (Table 4.3). This and other prognostic and predictive controversies are discussed further in chapter 7, which focuses on defining responses to TKI therapy and monitoring of patients.

In May 2011, Hasford and colleagues from the German CML group, proposed a new prognostic score, **Eu**ropean **T**reatment and **O**utcome **S**tudy (EUTOS) for CML that is heralded as being superior to the Sokal index and the Hasford score. The EUTOS score was based on capacity of clinical features at diagnosis to predict achievement of CCyR on imatinib. It requires only an

Table 4.3

Table 4.3
BCR–ABL1 Transcript Numbers at Three Months to Assess Response and Outcome in CML in Chronic Phase

Drug	Response @ 3 months	Level	Outcomes		Abstract[a]
Imatinib	Cytogenetics	CCyR	EFS	83% vs. 35%	3783, Latagliata
Imatinib	Molecular	≥10% IS	CCyR OS	91% vs. 47% 93% vs. 57%	1680, Milojkovic
Imatinib/ IFN-α	Molecular	≥10% IS	FFS EFS	94% vs. 86% 86% vs. 65%	1684, Nicolini
Imatinib	Molecular	≥10% IS	OS	97% vs. 87%	783, Hanfstein
Dasatinib	Molecular	≥10% IS	CCyR MMR CMR	93% vs. 76% 88% vs. 54% 20% vs. 0%	785, Marin

[a]Blood (ASH Annual Meeting Abstracts), Nov 2011; 118.

assessment of spleen size and percent basophils in blood. A formula $[0.0700 \times$ basophils $(\%) + 0.0402 \times$ spleen size (cm below LCM)] is then used and values >87 indicate high risk and <87 indicate low risk. Of 2060 patients in CCyR at 18 months following being on first-line treatment with imatinib, 211 were high risk and 1799 were low risk, the progression-free survival (PFS) was significantly better in the low-risk group versus the high-risk group (90% vs. 82%; $P = 0.006$) (Table 4.4).

It is of note that in 2012 the Hammersmith Hospital CML group attempted to validate the EUTOS score on a cohort of 277 consecutive patients with CML receiving imatinib as first-line therapy, and failed to significantly predict for the following outcomes: OS, PFS, CCyR, and MMR; conversely the Sokal score significantly predicted for all of these outcomes. Parenthetically, this observation appears not to have considered the notion of the EUTOS score being based on selecting patients for CCyR by 18 months. A similar unsuccessful validation of the EUTOS score was noted by the MDACC CML group. Regardless, the EUTOS score appears to be a relatively inexpensive tool which can help predict patients

Table 4.4
Prediction of Prognosis

	Sokal 1984	Euro 1998	EUTOS 2011
Parameters	Age	Age	
	Spleen	Spleen	Spleen
	Blasts	Blasts	
	Platelets	Platelets	
		Eosinophils	
		Basophils	Basophils
Treatment	Chemotherapy	Interferon	Imatinib
Endpoint	Survival	Survival	CCyR

who are likely to fare less well than expected and alternative therapies considered earlier and further independent validations must be sought.

"Be not the First by whom New Ways are Tried"
-Alexander Pope

Other parameters that appear to have some use as prognostic and predictive tools in the post–imatinib era, include functional aspects such as the import and export of the drug by influx and efflux pumps, respectively. Imatinib can be imported into cells by expression of human organic cation transporter type 1 (hOCT-1), and exported by ABCB1 and ABCG2. *In vitro* studies measuring imatinib uptake in mononuclear cells by hOCT-1 activity demonstrated that high OCT-1 activity was associated with higher response rates (in survival, EFS, molecular response, and mutation rate) compared with patients whose cells had low hOCT-1 activity. Other studies have suggested that hOCT-1 mRNA levels (which can be measured in a much easier and reproducible manner than imatinib uptake) also correlate with response. It is of interest that neither dasatinib nor nilotinib is transported by hOCT-1; rather, the activity of ABC efflux pumps may be involved in maintaining intracellular drug levels for these two TKIs.

The degree of myelosuppression, which an individual patient experiences on TKI may also be important. There is one multivariant analysis that supports the notion that patients who experience persistent grade 3 and 4 myelosuppression have an inferior response to TKI therapy with the lowest rates of CCyR. Other possible reasons for heterogeneity include variations in host and environmental factors and the epigenetic mechanisms in the CML cells, such as DNA methylation. Very recently investigators demonstrated that hypermethylation of the PDLIM4 gene is associated with shortened survival in patients with CML.

Current efforts have analyzed the potential use of genetic studies to help stratify patients into different risk categories. Molecular profiling of CD34+ cells has been noted to identify several genes, which are differentially expressed in low versus high-risk Sokal scores and could potentially be predictors of survival in patients with CML. By using gene expression profiling these and other investigators have been able to distinguish two subsets of patients: "aggressive," defined as those who developed blast transformation within three years of diagnosis, and "indolent" defined as those who entered blast transformation at least seven years following their initial diagnosis.

Several groups have also searched for genes associated with progression and resistance to TKI therapy in CML. Some of the preliminary findings suggest the presence of a robust gene "signature" of genes that are differentially expressed in advanced-phase disease compared with CP.

Where allogeneic SCT is being considered, Gratwohl and colleagues, on behalf of the European Group for Blood and Marrow Transplantation, have produced a risk-score based on pretransplant variables, which may predict the risk of mortality and relapse for patients treated by SCT. This was developed in 1997 based on a study of 3142 patients subjected to an allogeneic SCT in various phases of CML and remains useful in the current era (Fig. 4.8).

A gene-microarray–based risk score is currently being developed by Radich and colleagues, at the Fred Hutchinson Cancer

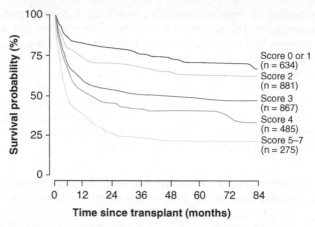

Figure 4.8
Allogeneic stem cell translplant risk: European Group for Blood and Marrow Transplantation scoring system. Source: From Gratwohl A, Hermans J, Goldman JM, et al. Risk assessment for patients with chronic myeloid leukaemia before allogeneic blood or marrow transplantation. Chronic Leukemia Working Party of the European Group for Blood and Marrow Transplantation. Lancet 1998; 352: 1087–92. A color version of this figure can be found in Plate IV *between pages 46 and 47.*

Center in Seattle, Washington, whereby a 6-gene signature could be used to predict relapse prior to allogeneic SCT for patients with CML in CP by integrating expert knowledge and gene expression data. Figure 4.9 depicts the methodology of integrating expert knowledge, predicted functional relationships, and microarray data to derive predictive genes that are biologically relevant to CML in CP and Figure 4.10 the signature genes (shown in orange) selected using the base reference genes (shown in pink) and weight threshold log(10) using the full CML progression microarray data.

CONCLUSION

The past two decades have witnessed an increasing proportion of patients with CML being diagnosed following a routine blood test and prior to the emergence of any clinical features. Many of these patients are in early-stage chronic phase. The introduction

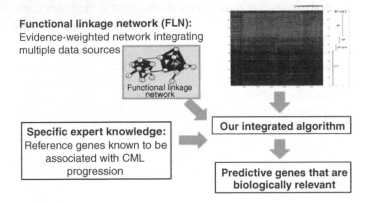

Functional linkage network (FLN):
Evidence-weighted network integrating multiple data sources

Functional linkage network

Specific expert knowledge:
Reference genes known to be associated with CML progression

Our integrated algorithm

Predictive genes that are biologically relevant

Figure 4.9
Predicting relapse prior to allogeneic stem cell translplant for patients with CML in chronic phase by integrating expert knowledge and gene expression data—an overview of the methodology. Abbreviation: *CML, chronic myeloid leukemia.* Source: *Courtesy of Professor Jerald Radich. A color version of this figure can be found in* Plate V *between pages 46 and 47.*

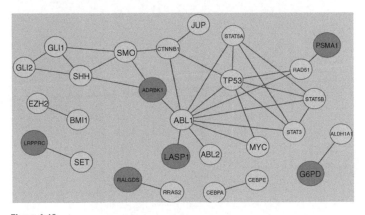

Figure 4.10
Predicting relapse prior to allogeneic stem cell translplant for patients with CML in chronic phase by integrating expert knowledge and gene expression data signature genes (●) selected using the base reference genes (○) and weight threshold log(10) using the full CML progression gene microarray data. Abbreviation: *CML, chronic myeloid leukemia.* Source: *Courtesy of Professor Jerald Radich.*

of imatinib appears to have changed not only the treatment paradigm for patients with CML but also the natural history of the disease. *Pari passu*, methods to stratify patients in accordance with the risks associated with disease and treatment-related parameters have improved. Notably prognostic scores in use during the pre–imatinib era have also been validated for current use. We can anticipate further advancements in the genetic applications and the identification and use of more robust candidate genes in the near future.

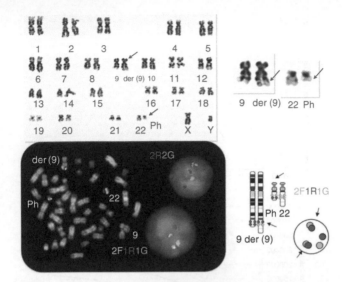

Figure 3.1
(i) Full and partial G banding of a Philadelphia (Ph) chromosome (+) cell (top) and
(ii) BCR–ABL1 positive metaphase and interphase cell with florescent in situ
hybridization (FISH) signals (2F1R1G) from D-FISH BCR–ABL1 probe (Vysis) along with
a normal interphase nucleus (2R2G) for comparison on the left and a cartoon explaining
the D-FISH pattern on the right (bottom half). Source: *Courtesy of Dr Ellie Nacheva.*

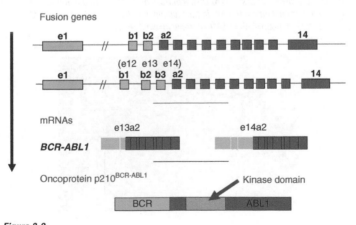

Figure 3.2
A schematic representation of the molecular anatomy of the Philadelphia (Ph) chromosome.

Plate I

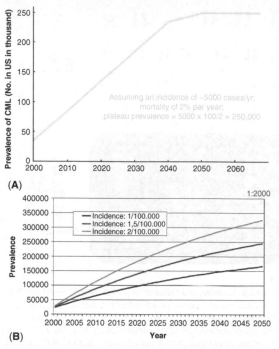

Figure 4.1
*Estimated prevalence of CML in (**A**) USA (courtesy of Professor Hagop Kantarjian); (**B**) Europe from Hehlmann R. CML in the imatinib era. Best Pract Res Clin Hematol 2009; 22: 283–4. Abbreviation: CML, chronic myeloid leukemia.*

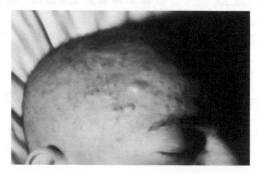

Figure 4.4
A patient with chronic myeloid leukemia in blast crisis and leukemia cutis.

Plate II

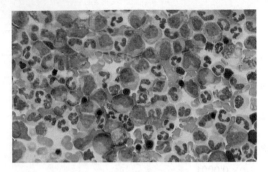

Figure 4.5
A photomicrograph of a peripheral blood film from a patient with chronic myeloid leukemia in chronic phase.

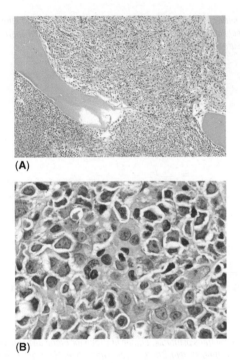

(A)

(B)

Figure 4.6
Photomicrographs of bone marrow biopsy from a patient with chronic myeloid leukemia in myeloid blast crisis (A) low and (B) high magnification.

Plate III

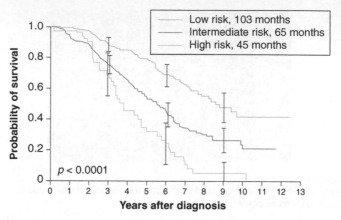

Figure 4.7
Probability of survival and median survival values for a population of chronic myeloid leukemia patients classified into low, intermediate, and high risk categories according to the Hasford (Euro) prognostic system (3).

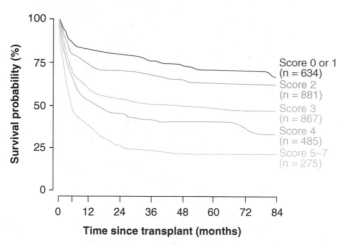

Figure 4.8
Allogeneic stem cell translplant risk: European Group for Blood and Marrow Transplantation scoring system. Source: From Gratwohl A, Hermans J, Goldman JM, et al. Risk assessment for patients with chronic myeloid leukaemia before allogeneic blood or marrow transplantation. Chronic Leukemia Working Party of the European Group for Blood and Marrow Transplantation. Lancet 1998; 352: 1087–92.

Plate IV

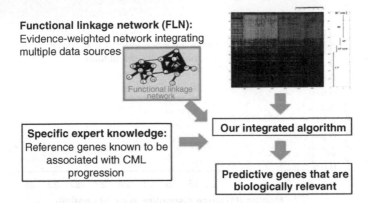

Functional linkage network (FLN): Evidence-weighted network integrating multiple data sources

Specific expert knowledge: Reference genes known to be associated with CML progression

Our integrated algorithm

Predictive genes that are biologically relevant

Figure 4.9
Predicting relapse prior to allogeneic stem cell translplant for patients with CML in chronic phase by integrating expert knowledge and gene expression data—an overview of the methodology. Abbreviation: *CML, chronic myeloid leukemia.* Source: *Courtesy of Professor Jerald Radich.*

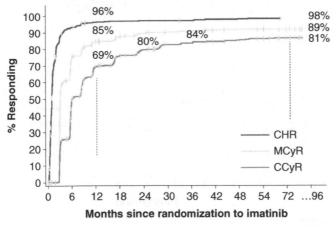

Figure 5.1
IRIS trial Kaplan–Meier estimates following eight years of follow-up. Abbreviations: *CCyR, complete cytogenetic response; CHR, complete hematologic response; IRIS, International Randomized Trial of Interferon-α with Cytarabine versus STI571; MCyR, major cytogenetic response.* Source: *Courtesy of Professor Michael Deininger, presented at ASH 2009.*

Plate V

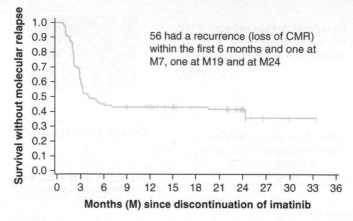

Figure 5.4
Preliminary Kaplan–Meier estimates of sustained CMR after discontinuation of imatinib from the French STIM study. Abbreviations: CMR, complete molecular response; STIM, Stop Imatinib. Source: From Mahon FX, Réa D, Guilhot J, et al. Discontinuation of imatinib in patients with chronic myeloid leukaemia who have maintained complete molecular remission for at least 2 years: the prospective, multicentre Stop Imatinib (STIM) trial. Lancet Oncol 2010; 11: 1029–35.

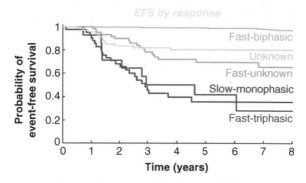

Figure 5.5
Mathematical models to assess BCR–ABL1 transcript dynamics: EFS according to patient group ($P < 0.0001$ for the comparison between fast-biphasic and all other categories). Abbreviation: EFS, event-free survival. Source: From Stein AM, Bottino D, Modur V, et al. BCR-ABL transcript dynamics support the hypothesis that leukemic stem cells are reduced during imatinib treatment. Clin Cancer Res 2011; 17: 6812–21.

Plate VI

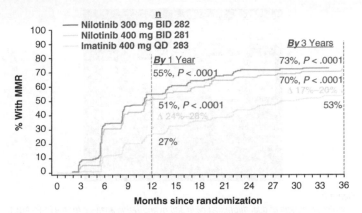

Figure 5.7
ENESTnd 36 months results—cumulative incidence of MMR. Abbreviations: ENESTnd,
Evaluating Nilotinib Efficacy and Safety in Clinical Trials-newly diagnosed patients;
MMR, major molecular response. Source: Courtesy of Professor Guiseppe Saglio,
presented at ASH 2011.

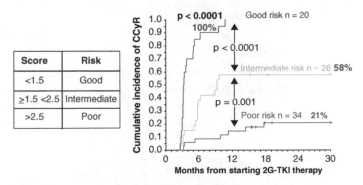

Figure 6.2
Hammersmith Hospital Score for predicting CCyR to second-generation TKIs.
Abbreviations: CCyR, complete cytogenetic response; TKIs, tyrosine kinase inhibitors.
Source: From Milojkovic D, Nicholson E, Apperley JF, et al. Early prediction of success
or failure of treatment with second-generation tyrosine kinase inhibitors in patients with
chronic myeloid leukemia. Haematologica 2010; 95: 224–31.

Plate VII

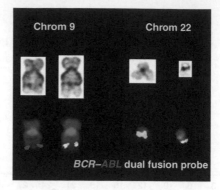

Figure 8.1
A photomicrograph of dual fluorescence in situ hybridization analysis for the BCR–ABL1 *fusion gene.*

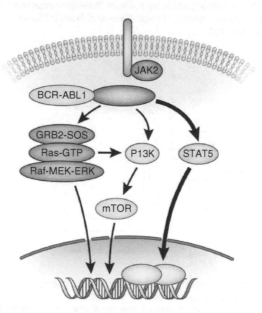

Figure 10.1
Schematic representation of STAT5 activation in Ph-positive chronic myeloid leukemia:
BCR–ABL1 phosphorylates STAT5 at the same critical tyrosine residue close to the
SH2 domain, inducing the same downstream events independently of JAK2.
Source: *Courtesy of Dr Doriano Fabbro.*

Plate VIII

5 Primary treatment of chronic myeloid leukemia

GENERAL PRINCIPLES

Since the introduction of imatinib, the "first generation," or the "original" tyrosine kinase inhibitor (TKI), into the clinic in 1998, the drug has become the preferred treatment for the majority, if not all, newly diagnosed patients with chronic myeloid leukemia (CML) in chronic phase (CP), except perhaps for children. Imatinib reduces substantially the number of CML cells in a patient's body, resulting in a complete hematologic response (CHR) in almost all such patients and a complete cytogenetic response (CCyR) in the vast majority (Fig. 5.1).

Imatinib has now significantly changed the prognosis of CML, and by 2009, an improvement in survival has been confirmed. With imatinib, the estimated 7- to 10-year survival is 80–85%, increasing to 90–93% if only CML-related deaths are considered (Fig. 1.3). Current experience suggests that about 2% of all CP patients progress to advanced phase disease each year, which contrasts with estimated annual progression rates of more than 15% for patients treated with hydroxycarbamide (previously known as hydroxyurea) and about 8–10% for patients receiving interferon-α (IFN-α), either with or without cytarabine.

Complete molecular responses (CMR) are, however, infrequent and then only after some years of treatment and probably in less than 50% of patients. It is therefore highly probable that imatinib will not eradicate residual CML in the vast majority of patients. A current central issue is therefore whether total eradication of all residual leukemia stem cells is actually necessary, because the

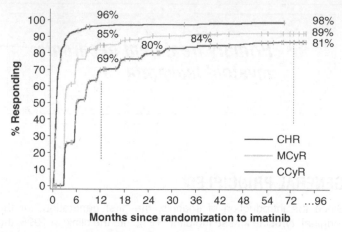

Figure 5.1
IRIS trial Kaplan–Meier estimates following eight years of follow-up. Abbreviations: CCyR, complete cytogenetic response; CHR, complete hematologic response; IRIS, International Randomized Trial of Interferon-α with Cytarabine versus STI571; MCyR, major cytogenetic response. Source: Courtesy of Professor Michael Deininger, presented at ASH 2009. A color version of this figure can be found in Plate V *between pages 46 and 47.*

survival of small numbers of residual leukemia stem cells might be compatible with long-term survival in an individual patient. This would be tantamount to cure at an operational level, as may well be the case after allogeneic stem cell transplantation (SCT). Allogeneic SCT was the preferred first-line therapy for patients with CML in CP in the pre–TKI era, but it is now reserved for those who do not achieve an optimal response on TKI, develop progressive disease on TKI, children, and in some parts of the world for economic reasons.

In this chapter, the current treatment algorithms for patients with CML are addressed, and some of the challenges for the future are speculated, in particular the use of the second-generation TKIs, dasatinib and nilotinib, for the treatment of newly diagnosed patients in the CP. Furthermore, the decision-making process might become complex when imatinib will become available in generic formulations in the next few years, at a significantly lower cost than the newly approved second-generation TKIs.

A POTENTIAL TREATMENT ALGORITHM FOR A NEWLY DIAGNOSED PATIENT WITH CML IN CHRONIC PHASE

Until the end of the 20th century, it was standard practice to recommend allogeneic SCT to all patients younger than 50 years with newly diagnosed CML in CP, provided they had suitable Human Leucocyte Antigen (HLA)-identical sibling or "HLA-matched" unrelated donors. For patients who were not considered suitable for an allogeneic SCT, or did not wish to proceed with it, were typically offered treatment with IFN-α alone or in combination with cytarabine. Patients presenting in the advanced phases of CML usually received combination chemotherapy, often followed by an allogeneic SCT if a "second" CP could be achieved.

The treatment algorithm for the newly diagnosed patients changed dramatically once the impressive success of imatinib in inducing CCyR in the vast majority of newly diagnosed patients with CML in CP was recognized. Thereafter, imatinib became the preferred first-line therapy worldwide. This is now challenged by the emerging data from the first-line studies with the second-generation TKIs, in particular dasatinib and nilotinib. Both of these drugs were granted regulatory approval in late 2010 in the USA and Switzerland, and now licensed in most other parts of the world. The preliminary results from the first-line use of bosutinib were also presented recently and did not meet the primary endpoint of the trial, and further follow-up is ongoing.

So How Have These Important Developments Affected the Potential Treatment Algorithm for a Newly Diagnosed Patient with CML in CP in 2012?

There is now general agreement that most new adult patients in the CP should first receive treatment with imatinib, dasatinib, or nilotinib. There are, perhaps, two exceptions to this general rule. First, some pediatricians feel that the results of allogeneic SCT in children are so comparatively good that it is reasonable to offer children with matched donors an allograft as initial treatment or after cytoreduction for a finite period with imatinib; neither dasatinib nor nilotinib has been tested adequately in children. Others feel that a child responding well to imatinib should be continued indefinitely on this agent. For treating children, there seems, at present, no general consensus.

The July 2011 report from the French National Phase IV trialists, in which 44 children (10 months to 17 years of age) with CML in CP were enrolled, confirmed imatinib's efficacy and safety profile to be similar to that in adults, but cautioned for a longer follow-up. Second, a case can be made for transplanting as initial therapy in patients for whom the cost of a TKI continued over many years would be totally prohibitive; this, of course, might change when imatinib will become available in generic formulations in the next few years. For such patients, a one-off procedure involving allogeneic SCT might be a better option. This is exemplified in many emerging countries where the cost of continuing TKI therapy on a long-term basis is simply prohibitive. Imatinib, for example, has an annual cost of about US$ 40,000, and with the increasing prevalence of CML, as a direct consequence of reduced mortality, the cost is compounded; an allogeneic SCT procedure in some of these countries (which can accord long-term remission to about 60% of the patients) can cost about US$ 40,000–50,000 or less.

For an adult, the question whether to start treatment with imatinib 400 mg/day or to embark on treatment with a second-generation TKI cannot currently be resolved. Tolerability appears to be the critical aspect in the high-dose trials with several investigators concluding that the lack of an overall benefit with the higher doses of imatinib may be due, at least in part, to the frequent dose reductions and treatment interruptions due to toxicity. This is further discussed in this chapter. Currently most specialists do not recommend higher starting doses outside of a clinical trial.

We have more than 10 years of experience with imatinib (at the standard dose of 400 mg daily) and over half of all patients appear to be doing remarkably well. We have only very limited experience with the use of the second-generation TKIs as initial therapy, but the preliminary results required by the US regulatory agency, with at least a 12-month follow-up, suggested that both nilotinib and dasatinib were superior to imatinib in terms of the achieving molecular and cytogenetic responses. Although superior responses with nilotinib are holding at 36 months analysis of the ENESTnd trial, the CCyR rate with dasatinib on the DASISION trial at 24 months may not be significantly different than in the imatinib arm, it is generally accepted that both drugs could replace imatinib as the preferred treatment for newly diagnosed patients with CML in CP. A further follow-up should help establish firmly the candidacy of either second-generation TKI to be used as frontline therapy. There is as yet no difference in progression-free survival (PFS) or overall survival (OS) in ENESTnd or DASI-SION between imatinib and the second-generation TKI arms.

The decision-making process is facilitated by optimizing monitoring response to therapy [cytogenetics, fluorescent-*insitu*-hybridization (FISH), molecular studies] by adopting guidelines such as those prepared by the European LeukemiaNet (ELN), which are discussed in chapter 7; a potential treatment algorithm is also depicted (Fig. 5.2), which undoubtedly will have evolved by the time this handbook is published!

With this caveat, most specialists today will commence a newly diagnosed adult patient on imatinib at 400 mg orally, once daily. Imatinib, a 2-phenylaminopyrimidine, was thought originally to act by occupying the ATP-binding pocket of the Abl kinase component of the BCR–ABL oncoprotein and thereby blocking the capacity of the enzyme to phosphorylate downstream effector molecules; it is now thought to act also by binding to an adjacent domain in a manner that holds the Abl component of the BCR–ABL1 oncoprotein molecule in an inactive configuration (Fig. 5.3). The drug rapidly reverses the clinical and hematological abnormalities and induces major cytogenetic responses (MCyR) in more than 80% of previously untreated chronic-phase patients.

The standard starting dose of initial imatinib is 400 mg/day, although several single-arm studies suggest that higher doses, up to 800 mg daily, might give better results with a greater proportion of patients achieving CCyR and major molecular response (MMR). Such studies

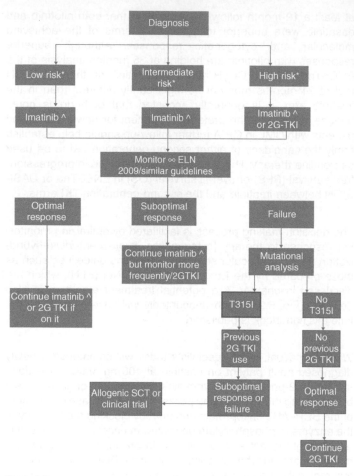

Figure 5.2

Potential treatment algorithm for a newly diagnosed patient with CML in CP. Abbreviations: CML, chronic myeloid leukemia; CP, chronic phase; ELN, European LeukemiaNet; SCT, stem cell transplant; 2G-TKI, second-generation tyrosine kinase inhibitor.

also suggest better PFS and transformation-free survival but with potentially more side effects, particularly myelosuppression. Some of the studies on higher dose imatinib are still ongoing, and until the longer-term results are available, it is reasonable to start newly diagnosed patients in CP on 400 mg daily (Table 5.1).

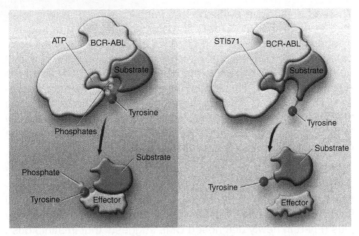

Figure 5.3
Mechanism of action of imatinib. Source: *From Goldman JM, Mughal TI. Chronic myeloid leukaemia. In: Hoffbrand AV, Catovsky D, Tuddenham EGD, Green AR, eds. Postgraduate Haematology 6E. Wiley, Chichester, 2010: 483–502.*

Table 5.1
Summary of Clinical Trials of Imatinib as Initial Therapy in Patients with CML in CP

Trial	n	Imatinib Dose (mg)	12 Months Response Rates
TOPS	476	400	CCyR 66%; MMR 40%
		800	CCyR 70% (NS); MMR 46%
GIMEMA/ELN	216	400	CCyR 58%; MMR 36%
		800	CCyR 64% (NS); MMR 43%(NS)
TIDEL-I	103	600/800	CCyR 88%; MMR 47%
French SPIRIT	319	400	CCyR 57%; MMR 40%
		600	CCyR 65%; MMR 52%
German CML IV	324	400	CCyR 50%; MMR 31%
	338	800	CCyR 63%; MMR 55%

Abbreviations: CCyR, complete cytogenetic response; CML, chronic myeloid leukemia; CP, chronic phase; ELN, European LeukemiaNet; GIMEMA, Gruppo Italiano Malattie Ematologiche dell'Adulto; MMR, major molecular response; NS, not statistically significant versus imatinib 400 mg daily arm; SPIRIT, STI571 prospective randomized trial; TIDEL, therapeutic intensification in de-novo leukemia; TOPS, tyrosine kinase inhibitor optimization and selectivity.

There is persuasive evidence that imatinib 600 mg daily is tolerated in more than 80% of CML patients and results in superior cytogenetic and molecular responses at 12 and 24 months compared with the conventional 400 mg daily dose, from the phase III French STI571 Prospective Randomized Trial (SPIRIT) and the Australian phase II Therapeutic Intensification in de novo Leukemia (TIDEL-I) trials. There are also several other trials, including the phase III Tyrosine Kinase Inhibitor Optimization and Selectivity (TOPS) and the phase III Gruppo Italiano Malattie Ematologiche dell'Adulto (GIMEMA) that failed to show benefit.

Interestingly, an April 2011 report from the German CML IV trialists on the results of the phase III study of tolerability-adapted imatinib 800 mg daily versus 400 mg daily versus 400 mg daily plus IFN-α in newly diagnosed CML suggests that imatinib dose can be optimized by a strategy that involves administering high-dose therapy early followed by an adjustment of the dose in accordance with individual patients' tolerance. Hehlmann and colleagues who conducted this study show that such an approach results in improving the proportion of patients who achieve MMR at 12 months. The superior responses with imatinib 800 mg daily remain so with a 36-month follow-up; the difference pertaining to CMR is even larger. The investigators of this trial explain this by the tolerability-adapted approach in the high-dose arm, which leads to a lower median dosage but a probably better compliance.

Much of what we have learned about the use of imatinib at the standard (400 mg daily) dose in first-line treatment of CML comes, remarkably, from a single international study. This was the prospective randomized phase III trial, known as the International Randomized Trial of Interferon Alfa with Cytarabine versus STI571 (IRIS), designed to compare imatinib as a single agent at a dose of 400 mg administered orally daily with the combination of IFN-α with cytarabine in previously untreated patients. It started recruitment in June 2000 and by January 2001, 1106 patients with untreated CML in CP had been recruited from 16 countries. Analysis after eight years of follow-up (December 2009; the last "formal" follow-up) showed that 55% of the patients who remained on imatinib therapy had achieved a CCyR (Table 5.2).

Table 5.2
Eight-Year Follow-Up Results of the IRIS Trial

Still on first-line imatinib	304 (55%)
Discontinued imatinib	249 (45%)
Adverse events/abnormal labs	30 (5.4%)
Suboptimal response	77 (13.9%)
Death	16 (2.9%)
SCT	16 (2.9%)
Withdrawal consent	44 (8%)
No reconsent to amendment	19 (3.4%)
Crossed over to IFN+Ara-C[a]	14 (2.5%)
Other reasons[b]	3 (6%)

[a]Due to intolerance (0.7%), lack of MCyR at 12 months or progression (1.8%).
[b]Includes administrative problems, protocol violation, lost to follow-up.
Abbreviations: IFN, interferon; IRIS, International Randomized Trial of Interferon Alfa with Cytarabine versus STI571; MCyR, major cytogenetic response; SCT, stem cell transplantation.

The cumulative best CCyR rate was 82% of all patients randomized to receive imatinib. The event-free survival (EFS) was 83% and the estimated OS was 93% (CML-related deaths) (Figs. 5.1 and 1.3). Furthermore, comparing survival in patients treated with imatinib with historical controls treated with IFN-α or IFN-α plus cytarabine provides strong support for the notion that the survival benefit is directly attributable to the improved cytogenetic response and is likely to be appreciable with imatinib. A substantial proportion of the patients in CCyR also achieved a MMR, and this proportion seems to have continued to increase steadily with time of imatinib; small minorities of patients achieve a CMR. The IRIS study also showed that 18% of imatinib-treated patients do not achieve a CCyR, and 10% who do will relapse; an additional 8% of patients were intolerant of imatinib.

The current safety analysis of imatinib is quite impressive, with very few potentially serious long-term effects. Side effects include nausea, headache, skin reactions, infraorbital edema, bone pains, and, sometimes, more generalized fluid retention. The skin reactions can from time to time be treated by temporarily interrupting imatinib and then reinstituting it under short-term corticosteroid cover. Hepatotoxicity characterized by raised serum transaminases is occasionally seen and may necessitate stopping the drug. There was initially concern about the potential for myocardial toxicity, but the updated (2009) IRIS trial analysis has confirmed that the risk is no higher than that of the normal population. There remains, however, a concern for the older patients who are anemic and may have preexisting cardiac disease. It is therefore appropriate to exercise caution under these circumstances (Table 5.3).

There has also been some concern about the potential to induce secondary malignancies, in particular myelodysplastic syndromes and acute myeloid leukemia (AML), and a small excess of urothelial tumors were reported in one small series. Other rare but potentially serious adverse effects of imatinib have included cerebral edema and excessive weight gain. Myelotoxicity appears to be dose related and reversible. When higher doses of imatinib are used, many patients require adjunctive therapy with myeloid growth factors, which can be given quite safely.

The concerns with regard to the precise definitions of response, in particular suboptimal response and monitoring, are addressed in

Table 5.3
Principal Short-Term Side Effects of Imatinib

Adverse Events Grade 1–2	% Patients	Adverse Events Grade 3–4	% Patients
Edema	60	Neutropenia	17
Muscle cramps	49	Thrombocytopenia	9
Diarrhea	45	Anemia	4
Nausea	50	LFT abnormalities	5
Musculoskeletal pain	47	Other	17
Rash/skin	40		
Abdominal pain	37		
Fatigue	39		
Joint pain	31		
Headache	37		

Abbreviation: LFT, Liver Function Tests.

chapter 7. It is, however, of some interest that the 2009 analysis of the IRIS cohort suggests that the actual time to achieve a CCyR does not appear to affect the long-term outcome. This is at variance with the current definitions of response, such as those proposed by the ELN, which consider anything less than a CCyR at 12 months to be suboptimal (Table 5.4).

The relationship between the level of residual disease and risk of disease progression is, however, well recognized. Patients who consistently attain a 3-log reduction in the concentration of *BCR–ABL1* transcripts, compared with the baseline, appear to have a lower risk of disease progression compared with those who attain lesser degrees of molecular responses.

Can Imatinib Therapy Ever be Discontinued?

The challenge of how long to continue imatinib remains unresolved. For the patient who has achieved a CCyR, stopping the drug usually leads to recurrence of Ph positivity and eventually leukocytosis in the majority of cases, although, on occasion, the cytogenetic remission continues without treatment for many months or even longer. The best effort, so far, in addressing this unresolved challenge comes from the French Stop Imatinib (STIM) study led by Mahon and colleagues in Bordeaux. They observed that a small proportion of the patients who achieved a CMR

Table 5.4
Potential Long-Term Side Effects of Imatinib

- Cardiac toxicities
- Secondary malignancies
- Myositis
- Renal failure
- Dermatitis
- Pancreatitis
- Hypophosphatemia
- Gynecomastia
- Hypogammaglobinemia opportunistic infections
- Endocrinopathies
- Weight gain

(equivalent to a >4-log reduction in *BCR–ABL1* transcript numbers; Table 7.2) that lasted more than two years have stopped taking imatinib and though some subsequently relapsed, others did not (Fig. 5.4). Importantly, all patients who had a molecular relapse responded promptly to the reintroduction of imatinib, suggesting that discontinuation did not result in an acquired resistance.

This interesting observation raises the possibility that imatinib may have the capacity to eradicate CML in some cases, and not other. The STIM study identified patients with a low Sokal risk score, male gender, and longer duration of imatinib treatment as potential prognostic factors for the maintenance of CMR after discontinuing imatinib. At present, the best advice for the responding patient is to continue the drug indefinitely.

The recent work by Stein and colleagues using mathematical models of *BCR–ABL1* levels to assess the dynamics of CML stem cells is of considerable interest in this regard. They did this by testing

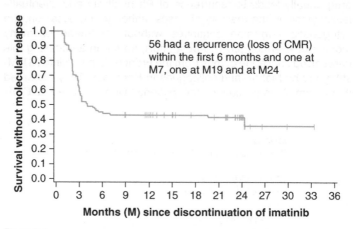

Figure 5.4
Preliminary Kaplan–Meier estimates of sustained CMR after discontinuation of imatinib from the French STIM study. Abbreviations: CMR, complete molecular response; STIM, Stop Imatinib. Source: From Mahon FX, Réa D, Guilhot J, et al. Discontinuation of imatinib in patients with chronic myeloid leukaemia who have maintained complete molecular remission for at least 2 years: the prospective, multicentre Stop Imatinib (STIM) trial. Lancet Oncol 2010; 11: 1029–35. A color version of this figure can be found in Plate VI *between pages 46 and 47.*

three potential scenarios: (*i*) monoexponential, in which there is no or very little decline in *BCR–ABL1* transcripts; (*ii*) biexponential, in which patients have a rapid initial decrease in *BCR–ABL1* transcripts followed by a more gradual response; and (*iii*) triexponential, in which patients first exhibit a biphasic decline but then have a third phase when *BCR–ABL1* transcripts increase rapidly. They found that most patients treated with imatinib exhibit a biphasic decrease in *BCR–ABL1* transcript levels, with a rapid decrease during the first few months of treatment, followed by a more gradual decrease that often continues over many years (Fig. 5.5). Based on this, they speculate why some patients are unable to discontinue imatinib therapy without relapse.

Efforts by Tessa Holyoake in Glasgow and others have, of course, shown *in vitro* evidence that CML stem cells are resistant to imatinib and the second-generation TKIs (Fig. 5.6). In March 2012, Chomel and colleagues in Poitiers, France, demonstrated substantial lower *BCR–ABL1* expression in the CML progenitors and primitive stem cells. They speculate that these low levels of *BCR–ABL1* expression could be an additional mechanism for TKI resistance and if so, the use of more potent TKIs is unlikely to

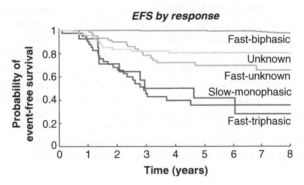

EFS by response

Figure 5.5
Mathematical models to assess BCR–ABL1 transcript dynamics: EFS according to patient group (P < 0.0001 for the comparison between fast-biphasic and all other categories). Abbreviation: EFS, event-free survival. Source: From Stein AM, Bottino D, Modur V, et al. BCR-ABL transcript dynamics support the hypothesis that leukemic stem cells are reduced during imatinib treatment. Clin Cancer Res 2011; 17: 6812–21. A color version of this figure can be found in Plate VI between pages 46 and 47.

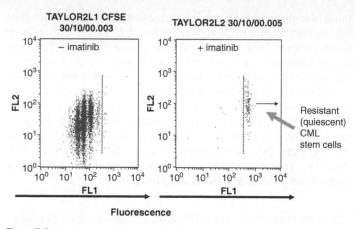

Figure 5.6
CML stem cells are resistant to imatinib. Abbreviation: CML, chronic myeloid leukemia. Source: Courtesy of Professor Tessa Holyoake.

abrogate this. Rather, alternative therapies would be required to eradicate the persistent CML stem cells.

Clearly it is simply not feasible for some individuals, such as pregnant patients, to continue imatinib indefinitely. A transatlantic series by Pye and colleagues in 2008 identified fetal abnormalities in 12 of 125 evaluable pregnancies. The abnormalities ranged from premature closure of skull sutures (craniosynostosis), hypoplastic lungs, exomphalos (omphalocele), renal abnormalities, and skeletal anomalies. Other smaller series have also suggested increased risk of birth defects and spontaneous abortions in women taking the drug throughout pregnancy. Women of childbearing age should therefore be offered adequate contraception while on imatinib. Currently, it is best to adhere similar advice for the use of second-generation TKIs.

A topical question is how the use of imatinib in men might affect pregnancy outcomes. Approximately 60 pregnancies have been reported in partners of men on imatinib. There are no suggestions of any problems in conception, pregnancy, delivery, or of any increase in congenital abnormalities. An anecdotal report of one family with two sons affected by same abnormality has been described.

An alternative treatment option for the small minority of newly diagnosed patients in CP that would benefit from an immediate allogeneic SCT compared with continuing imatinib irrespective of the outcome from imatinib has been tested in a retrospective analysis from the Center for International Blood and Marrow Transplant Research (CIBMTR) and the European Group for Blood and Marrow Transplantation (EBMT). It suggests that for adult patients, including those with low risk for transplant-related mortality by EBMT criteria, it is not possible to identify a cohort who would clearly benefit from an immediate allogeneic SCT versus continuing imatinib irrespective of the outcome from imatinib. The outcome for children, those with a potential syngeneic donor and possibly those with high-risk disease by Sokal or Hasford criteria, is uncertain. The current EBMT recommendations, however, suggest that patients with high-risk disease and a low-transplant risk should probably still be considered for an early allogeneic SCT. Such a cohort, if treated with imatinib in the first instance, should probably not receive a second-generation TKI on relapse (see below) and rather proceed to allogeneic SCT.

The MDACC group reported in March 2011 that an early allogeneic SCT should be considered for patients who appear to have a low probability of responding to a second-generation TKI, in particular those who harbor BCR–ABL1 point mutations. With regard to children, some pediatric hematologists still recommend initial treatment by allogeneic SCT for patients younger than 16 years who have HLA-identical siblings, largely because of a lack of adequate data pertaining to the use of safety of imatinib as first-line therapy in children, as discussed above.

Second-Generation TKIs as Potential First-Line Therapy for Patients with CML in Chronic Phase

Dasatinib

Dasatinib is an oral dual kinase inhibitor that entered the clinics in 2003. It is a smaller thiazole-carboxamide molecule than imatinib to which it bears little chemical relationship. Unlike imatinib, dasatinib appears to inhibit the enzymatic activity of the BCR–ABL1 oncoprotein regardless of the position of the BCR–ABL1 activation loop, and it targets a much wider range of tyrosine kinases. It also inhibits some of the SRC family kinases. Preclinical studies showed that dasatinib was 300-fold more potent than imatinib.

Following the success in the treatment of patients with CML in CP resistant/refractory or intolerant to imatinib, the drug was approved for the treatment of all phases of CML with intolerance or resistance/refractoriness to imatinib and all patients with Ph-positive ALL. Dasatinib was noted to overcome most mechanisms of resistance to imatinib, with the exception of the T315I mutation.

The drug thereafter entered an international randomized phase III trial comparing it with imatinib for frontline therapy of newly diagnosed patients with CML in CP. A total of 519 such patients were recruited into the Dasatinib versus Imatinib Study in Treatment-Naïve CML Patients (DASISION) trial, and the initial results were published in June 2010 and the updated results, following a median follow-up of 24 months, published in February 2012.

At the time of latest analysis, 199 (77%) dasatinib-treated patients and 194 (75%) imatinib-treated patients remained on study; more patients required dose interruptions among those treated with dasatinib (59%) compared with those receiving imatinib (43%). The median dose intensities were 99.5 mg/day for dasatinib and 400 mg/day for imatinib. However, the rates of cumulative CCyR were superior in those patients receiving dasatinib therapy, both at 12 (85% vs. 73%) and at 24 months (86% vs. 82%); the cumulative CCyR rate was higher for dasatinib versus imatinib across the period analyzed ($P = 0.0002$; Table 5.5) At three months, CCyR rates were 54% with dasatinib versus 31% with imatinib, increasing to 73% versus 59%, respectively, at six months; the median time to CCyR was 3.2 months for the dasatinib-treated patients, compared with 6.0 months for the imatinib-treated cohort. MMR rates by 12 and 24 months were significantly higher with dasatinib compared with imatinib (46% and 64% vs. 28% and 46%, respectively; $P < 0.0001$). Among the subgroup of patients who achieved MMR, median time to MMR was 15 months for dasatinib and 36 months for imatinib. CMR (defined in this study as a 4.5-log reduction in the *BCR–ABL1* transcripts, compared with baseline) was achieved in 17% of dastinib and 8% of imatinib-treated patients ($P = 0.002$).

Table 5.5

Current Results of Clinical Trials of Dasatinib and Nilotinib as Initial Therapy in CML in CP

						Response Rates (Intention to treat)							
			12 months			24 months			36 months			
Trial	N	CCyR	MMR	CMR	CCyR	MMR	CMR	CCyR	MMR	CMR			
DASISION[a]													
Dasatinib	258	85%	46%	NA	85%	64%	17%	NA	NA	NA			
Imatinib	258	73%	28%	NA	82%	46%	8%	NA	NA	NA			
ENESTnd[b]													
Nilotinib (300)	282	65%	55%	11%	87%	71%	26%	NA	73%	32%			
Nilotinib (400)	281	55%	51%	7%	85%	67%	21%	NA	70%	28%			
Imatinib	283	22%	27%	1%	77%	44%	10%	NA	53%	15%			

[a]DASISION trial: From Kantarjian HM, Shah NP, Cortes JE, et al. Dasatinib or imatinib in newly diagnosed chronic-phase chronic myeloid leukemia: 2-year follow-up from a randomized phase 3 trial (DASISION). Blood 2012; 119: 1123–9.
[b]ENESTnd trial: Saglio G et al., ASH meeting abstracts, 2011.

Abbreviations: CCyR, complete cytogenetic response; CML, chronic myeloid leukemia; CP, chronic phase; CMR, complete molecular response (4.5 log); DASISION, Dasatinib versus Imatinib Study in Treatment-Naïve CML Patients; ENESTnd, Evaluating Nilotinib Efficacy and Safety in Clinical Trials-newly diagnosed patients; MMR, major molecular response; N, number of patients; NA, not applicable.

Following a minimum follow-up of 24 months, transformation to the advanced phases of the disease was noted in 2.3% of the dasatinib and 5.0% of the imatinib-treated cohorts. In patients who discontinued therapy, BCR–ABL1 kinase domain mutational analysis confirmed the presence of mutations in 10 patients, in each arm.

Therapy was well tolerated with both TKIs, with grade 3–4 nonhematologic drug-related toxicities occurring in ≤1%. Fourteen percent of patients treated with dasatinib, compared with none treated with imatinib, developed pleural effusion, but only five (1.9%) discontinued therapy for such toxicity. The rates of fluid retention, superficial edema, myalgia, vomiting, and rash were more common with imatinib, whereas the rates of diarrhea, fatigue, and headache were similar for both treatments. Drug-related pulmonary hypertension was noted in three (1.2%) dasatinib-treated patients, although in one patient, no evidence of pulmonary arterial hypertension was found on right heart catheterization; none of these three patients discontinued dasatinib. Seventeen dasatinib-treated patients (6.6%) and 14 imatinib-treated patients (5.4%) were reported to have a drug-related cardiac event.

Biochemical adverse events led to the discontinuation of four imatinib- and one dasatinib-treated patients. The principal abnormality was hypophosphatemia, which was of grade 3–4 hypophosphatemia in 7% of dasatinib and 25% of imatinib-treated patients. Rates of grade 3–4 anemia (11% vs. 8%) and neutropenia (24% vs. 21%) were similar, but more patients treated with dasatinib developed grade 3–4 thrombocytopenia compared with those treated with imatinib (19% vs. 11%).

Overall, the results reported by the DASISION studies suggest that first-line therapy with dasatinib renders higher response rates with a comparable toxicity profile compared with imatinib by 24 months of minimum follow-up. These observations have now been confirmed in the 36-month follow-up of the DASISION trial which was presented at the December 2012 American Society of Hematology (ASH) meeting. It remains unknown whether these higher rates of early response will translate into improved EFS and/or OS rates. Thus far, no differences in OS have been observed between the dasatinib (97%) and the imatinib (99%) arms. It is of note that although the cumulative CCyR rates for dasatinib versus imatinib have narrowed from 12% by 12 months (85% vs. 73%) to 4% by 24 months (86% vs. 82%), the difference in cumulative MMR rates seen by 12 months of 18% (46% vs. 28%) has remained consistent by 24 months (64% vs. 46%). Finally, it is of considerable interest that a CMR was observed in 17% of the dasatinib-treated patients compared with 8% of the imatinib-treated cohort. Dasatinib is currently approved for the first-line treatment of newly diagnosed patients with CML in CP by the US Food and Drug Administration (FDA), the EMEA, and several other countries but is not currently approved by the National Institute for Health and Clinical Excellence (NICE) in the UK.

Nilotinib

Nilotinib is an oral drug designed as a chemical modification of imatinib and similar to its precursor has a relatively narrow spectrum of activity against kinases other than Abl1, but *in vitro* approximately 30–50 times more potent. It, similar to imatinib, works by binding to a closed (inactive) conformation of the ABL1 KD, but with a much higher affinity. Similar to imatinib, it inhibits the dysregulated tyrosine kinase activity by occupying the ATP-binding pocket of the ABL1 kinase component of the BCR–ABL1 oncoprotein and blocking the capacity of the enzyme to phosphorylate downstream effector molecules. Nilotinib is also active in 32 of the currently 33 imatinib-resistant cell lines with mutant ABL1 kinases but has no activity against the T315I mutation.

It entered the clinics in 2004 and following confirmation of its safety and efficacy profile in patients who were either resistant or intolerant to imatinib, the drug was evaluated in the frontline use in patients with CML in CP. The ENESTnd trial is a phase III, randomized, open-label, multicenter study comparing the efficacy and safety of nilotinib with imatinib (Table 5.5). Eight hundred forty-six patients with CML in CP were randomly assigned 1:1:1 to nilotinib 300 mg twice daily ($n = 282$), nilotinib 400 mg twice daily ($n = 281$), or imatinib 400 mg/day ($n = 283$). The primary endpoint was MMR at 12 months, and patients were stratified by Sokal index, which resulted in equal distributions of low, intermediate, and high Sokal indexes in each arm of the trial. The initial results were published in June 2010 and the updated results, following a minimum follow-up of 24 months, published in September 2011.

More recently, the updated results following a minimum follow-up of 36 months were presented at the December 2011 ASH annual meeting (Fig. 5.7). Responses are not only more rapidly achieved with nilotinib, but all efficacy endpoints continue to be superior for nilotinib in the longer and updated follow-ups more recently reported. In particular, new progressions to AP/BP were not observed in the third year of treatment, and the differences between the number of progressions observed in both nilotinib arms were significantly lower with respect to those observed in the imatinib arm and remain significant not only for patients still in the core study (P = 0.0059, nilotinib 300 mg BID vs. imatinib; P = 0.0185, nilotinib 400 mg BID vs. imatinib) but also including those patients who discontinued from the study, in an intention to treat analysis (P = 0.0496, nilotinib 300 mg BID vs. imatinib; P = 0.0086, nilotinib 400 mg BID vs. imatinib).

Although a statistically significant OS advantage has not been so far observed for nilotinib- versus imatinib-treated patients; however, the deaths due to CML progressions are significantly lower in both nilotinib arms (P = 0.0356, nilotinib 300 mg BID vs. imatinib;

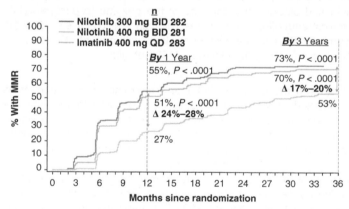

Figure 5.7
ENESTnd 36 months results—cumulative incidence of MMR. Abbreviations: ENESTnd, Evaluating Nilotinib Efficacy and Safety in Clinical Trials-newly diagnosed patients; MMR, major molecular response. Source: Courtesy of Professor Guiseppe Saglio, presented at ASH 2011. A color version of this figure can be found in Plate VII between pages 46 and 47.

P = 0.0159, nilotinib 400 mg BID vs. imatinib), and this is also due to the fact that the median survival of patients who progress at present is still less than one year (10.5 months). The cumulative rates of MMR were significantly higher for nilotinib 300 mg twice daily (73%, *P* < 0.0001) and nilotinib 400 mg twice daily (70%, *P* < 0.0001) than for imatinib (53%).

More patients achieved CMR[4.5] with nilotinib 300 mg twice daily (32%; *P* < 0.0001) and nilotinib 400 mg twice daily (28%; *P* = 0.0004) than with imatinib (15%). In patients who discontinued therapy, the number of patients with emerging mutations in the nilotinib group was about half that reported with imatinib treatment, and there were no major differences in the frequency of T315I mutations in either of the study cohorts.

In general, therapy was well tolerated in all the study cohorts, and treatment discontinuation due to adverse events was observed in 8%, 12%, and 10% of patients on nilotinib 300 mg twice daily, nilotinib 400 mg twice daily, and imatinib, respectively. Grade 3–4 thrombocytopenia was more common with nilotinib, compared with imatinib; in contrast, the imatinib-treated patients experienced more neutropenia (imatinib 21% vs. nilotinib 300 mg twice daily 12% and nilotinib 400 mg twice daily 11%). Grade 3–4 biochemical abnormalities with nilotinib, such as elevated levels of lipase, alanine aminotransferase, aspartate aminotransferase, total bilirubin, and glucose, were seen less often than those reported in earlier phase II nilotinib studies; two patients, however, discontinued the study due to acute pancreatitis: one in the imatinib group and one in the nilotinib 400 mg twice daily group.

There were no occurrences of corrected QTc interval by Fridericia's formula (QTcF) prolongation > 500 milliseconds in any of the study cohorts, although four patients in the nilotinib 300 mg twice daily group developed arrythmias and QTcF prolongation, considered not to be clinically relevant, by the investigators. Six patients were also reported to have had a peripheral arterial occlusive disease event within 24 months of follow-up, three (1%) in each nilotinib group. Notably, all six of these events occurred in patients with preexisting risk factors for the disease and only one of these events was judged to be related to the study drug by the investigator. Other grade 3–4 toxicities were reported in <1% of the study patients, with the exception of rash, 3% with nilotinib 400 mg twice daily and 2% with imatinib, and headache, 3% with nilotinib 300 mg twice daily and 1% with nilotinib 400 mg twice daily. Figure 5.8 depicts a Forest plot comparing differences in rates of drug-related nonhematologic and grade 3–4 hematologic adverse events for patients treated with nilotinib or imatinib.

Following a minimum follow-up of 36 months, the cumulative rates of MMR appear to increase for all groups of patients but remain significantly higher for the nilotinib- versus imatinib-treated patients: nilotinib 300 mg twice daily (73% (P < 0.001), nilotinib 400 mg twice daily (70% (P < 0.001), and imatinib (53%). It is noteworthy that with the recent 36 months safety update, there appears to be no significant changes in the toxicity of either dose of nilotinib or imatinib.

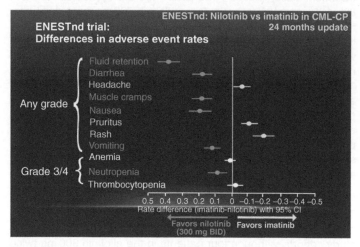

Figure 5.8
Forest plot comparing differences in adverse events rates for nilotinib and imatinib (ENESTnd trial). Abbreviation: ENESTnd, Evaluating Nilotinib Efficacy and Safety in Clinical Trials-newly diagnosed patients. Source: From Hochhaus A, Saglio G, le Coutre P, et al. Superior efficacy of nilotinib compared with imatinib in newly diagnosed patients with chronic myeloid leukemia in chronic (CML-CP); ENESTnd minimum 24-month follow-up. Haematologica 2011; 96: 203–4.

Overall, it is clear that nilotinib, at either dose, continues to show better efficacy than imatinib for the treatment of patients with newly diagnosed CML in CP. These results support nilotinib as a first-line treatment option for patients with newly diagnosed disease. Nilotinib at 300 mg twice daily, and not 400 mg twice daily, was approved for first-line use by the FDA and Switzerland in September 2010 and thereafter by EMEA and NICE; parenthetically, the later approval for the UK required the manufacturer (Novartis) to offer the drug at a considerably discounted National Health Service price.

TREATMENT OF PATIENTS WITH CML IN ADVANCED PHASE

The introduction of TKIs, in particular dasatinib, for the treatment of patients with CML in advanced phase has improved the response rates and the prognosis of these patients, particularly those in the accelerated phase. Historically, these patients have fared poorly and long-term remission could only be accorded to a small minority of patients who were suitable for an allogeneic SCT. Single-agent imatinib accorded a modest degree of success in this setting, but most patients still succumb to the disease due to lack of response and development of resistance, in particular due to kinase domain mutations. Studies of high-dose imatinib have shown a trend toward better cytogenetic response rates, but again these tend to be short-lived. Combinations of imatinib or, more recently, the second-generation TKI, dasatinib, with cytotoxic chemotherapy has proven to be more effective in managing patients. Dasatinib, in contrast to imatinib and nilotinib, is able to cross the blood–brain barrier and may afford an advantage compared with other TKIs regarding the prevention of central nervous system relapse, which is not uncommon in patients with lymphoid blast crisis. Moreover, studies from Van Etten Laboratory in Boston suggest that the SRC kinase inhibitory properties of dasatinib may have a role in the responses of patients with Ph-positive B-ALL.

Accelerated Phase Disease

At present, it is difficult to make general statements about the optimal management of patients in accelerated-phase disease, partly because the definition of this phase is not universally agreed.

Patients who have not previously been treated with imatinib may obtain benefit from the use of this agent. For patients who progressed to accelerated phase while on imatinib, it is best to discontinue imatinib and consider alternative strategies. More recent results from dasatinib monotherapy studies accord a higher success and the drug, at the higher dose of 70 mg twice daily, should be considered. Patients whose disease seems to be moving toward overt blast crisis may benefit from cytotoxic drug combinations appropriate for *de novo* AML or ALL.

Allogeneic SCT should certainly be considered for younger patients if suitable donors can be identified. A nonrandomized study from Peking University People's Hospital, published in March 2011, assessed the benefits of imatinib versus allogeneic SCT for 132 patients with CML in accelerated phase. The authors observed that SCT conferred a significant survival benefit for high- and intermediate-risk patients, compared with imatinib. Reduced intensity conditioning allografts are probably not indicated because the efficacy of the graft-versus-leukemia effect in advanced-phase CML is not established. Clinical trials exploring the use of either dasatinib or nilotinib should be considered, and the preliminary results, discussed above, are encouraging.

Blast Crisis

Patients in blast crisis may be treated with combinations of cytotoxic drug combinations analogous to those used for de novo AML or ALL, in the hope of prolonging life, but cure can no longer be a realistic objective. Based on preliminary experience with Ph-postive ALL, the usefulness of combining conventional cytotoxic drugs with TKI is now being explored. Patients in lymphoid transformation tend to fare slightly better in the short term than those in myeloid transformation. If intensive therapy is not deemed appropriate, one can offer a relatively innocuous drug such as hydroxyurea at higher than usual dosage; the blast cell numbers will be reduced substantially in most cases, but their numbers usually increase again within three to six weeks.

Combination chemotherapy may restore 20% of patients to a situation resembling chronic-phase disease, and this benefit may last for three to six months. A very small minority, probably less than 10%, may achieve substantial degrees of Ph-negative hematopoiesis. This is most likely in patients who entered blast crisis very soon after diagnosis. Imatinib can be remarkably effective in controlling the clinical and hematological features of CML in advanced phases in the very short term. In some patients in established myeloid blast crisis who received imatinib 600 mg/day, massive splenomegaly was entirely reversed and blast cells were eliminated from the blood and marrow, but such responses are almost always short-lived. Therefore imatinib, or if dasatinib is available, should be incorporated into a program of therapy that involves also the use of conventional cytotoxic drugs and possibly also allogeneic SCT. As in the case of accelerated-phase disease, it is useful to consider patients who enter blast crisis while on imatinib for clinical trials.

Allogeneic SCT using HLA-matched sibling donors can be performed in accelerated phase; the probability of leukemia-free survival at five years is 30–50%. Allogeneic SCT performed in overt blast crisis is nearly always unsuccessful. The mortality resulting from graft-versus-host disease is extremely high, and the probability of relapse in those who survive the transplant procedure is very considerable. The probability of survival at five years is consequently less than 10%.

CONCLUSION

The substantial understanding of the molecular features and pathogenesis of CML has provided important insights into targeting the treatment to specific molecular defects.

The successful introduction of imatinib, followed by dasatinib and nilotinib, as targeted therapy for CML has made the approach to management of the newly diagnosed patient fairly complex. Imatinib unequivocally established the principle that molecularly targeted treatment can work and the second-generation TKIs, dasatinib and nilotinib, appear to be more effective in terms of achieving a faster CCyR and MMR, but the follow-up period is still relatively short. There is, however, little doubt that both drugs appear to be more efficacious than imatinib in the first-line use,

Table 5.6

Arguments for and Against the Use of Second-Generation TKI as First-Line Therapy for CML in CP

Arguments in favor
- One-year response rates clearly better than with imatinib 400 mg/day
- Fewer failures in first year of treatment
- Incidence of failure seems to be lower at 2 yr than with imatinib

Arguments against
- 50–60% of patients will never need anything more than imatinib
- Well-defined and manageable toxicity
- Definitely cheaper

Abbreviations: CML, chronic myeloid leukemia; CP, chronic phase; TKI, tyrosine kinase inhibitor.

and the current safety analysis appears to suggest the notion that these drugs appear to be at least as safe for use as first-line therapy. Furthermore, both drugs appear to accord CMR, an emerging endpoint for discontinuing TKI therapy safely (see above), to a greater proportion of patients. The treatment algorithm for a newly diagnosed patient with CML-CP can therefore be anticipated to evolve substantially with a longer follow-up period for the second-generation TKIs. In Table 5.6, Professor John Goldman and I summarize some arguments that can be made for and against using these drugs as first-line treatment for most, if not all, newly diagnosed patients.

6 Secondary treatment and stem cell transplantation for chronic myeloid leukemia

Current experience with the use of imatinib as primary therapy suggests that up to a third of all patients with chronic myeloid leukemia (CML) in chronic phase, and significantly more in the advanced phase will require an alternative therapy within the first two years of treatment. The long-term data following the use of a second-generation tyrosine kinase inhibitor (TKI), dasatinib or nilotinib, for first-line therapy are not known at the present time, but the failure, although not necessarily the tolerance, is generally anticipated to be lower than that experienced with imatinib, but we cannot be sure at this time. It is, of course, of great clinical interest that the current results from randomized trials suggest better outcomes with both dasatinib and nilotinib, compared with standard dose imatinib, in particular the rates of major molecular responses (MMRs) and the event-free survival (EFS). Thus far, no differences in overall survival (OS) have been observed with either dasatinib or nilotinib.

A POTENTIAL TREATMENT ALGORITHM FOR A PATIENT WITH CML IN CHRONIC PHASE WHO IS RESISTANT OR INTOLERANT TO IMATINIB

Intolerance to imatinib occurs in about 10%, but resistance, both primary and secondary, is being increasingly recognized in a significant minority of patients in chronic phase. About 30% of patients with CML in chronic phase eventually become resistant to imatinib. Resistance is more common in patients who start imatinib in late chronic phase and advanced phase and is discussed in chapter 8. It occurs in about 70% of patients treated in myeloid blast crisis and in almost all of the patients in lymphoid blast crisis.

The majority of patients who are resistant/intolerant to imatinib should receive either dasatinib or nilotinib, both of which are approved for this indication in many parts of the world. Current experience with dasatinib in patients with CML in chronic phase resistant/refractory to imatinib suggests that about 90% of patients have a complete hematological response and 52% of patients have a complete cytogenetic response (CCyR). About 25% of patients with the more advanced phases of CML and Ph-positive acute lymphoblastic leukemia (ALL) also have reasonable responses. Responses are seen in patients with most of the currently known ABL kinase domain (KD) mutations, except the T315I mutation (also known as the "gatekeeper" mutation). Hematological toxicity is common, particularly in those with the advanced phases of CML and Ph-positive ALL. These include neutropenia (49%), thrombocytopenia (48%), and anemia (20%). Nonhematological toxicity includes diarrhea, headaches, superficial edema, pleural effusions, and occasional pericardial effusions. Grade 3/4 side effects are rare and grade 3/4 pleural effusions occurred in 6% of patients. The prospective randomized dasatinib dose optimization study confirmed the notion that a lower dose of dasatinib (100 mg daily) was as effective as the previously approved higher dose (70 mg twice daily) in terms of the hematological, and major and complete cytogenetic responses, including the time to achieve these responses, but the toxicity profile confirmed a much lower incidence of pleural and pericardial effusions. Following this, the approved dose of dasatinib for patients with CML in chronic phase was adjusted to 100 mg daily.

Current experience with nilotinib in patients with CML in chronic phase resistant or intolerant to imatinib suggests a complete hematological response of about 70% and a CCyR of about 40%. Patients in the advanced phases of CML also respond but to a lesser degree. The most common treatment-related toxicity is myelosuppression, followed by headaches, pruritus, and rashes. Overall, 22% of the patients experienced thrombocytopenia, with 19% having either grade 3 or 4 severity; 16% had neutropenia and a further 16% had anemia. Most of the nonhematological side effects were of a grade 1/2 severity. All including the hematological effects were fully reversible. About 19% of all patients experience arthralgias and about 14% experience fluid retention, particularly pleural and pericardial effusions. Importantly, patients with the imatinib-acquired T315I mutation appear to be refractory to nilotinib.

Until recently, it was less clear whether the responses accorded by these second-generation TKIs in imatinib-resistant or imatinib-intolerant patients were durable. In December 2011, the Hammersmith Group published a report confirming the durability of these responses, based on an intention to treat analysis of 119 consecutive patients (including three who received bosutinib). The four-year probabilities of OS and EFS were 81.9% and 35.3%, respectively. To assess the durability of cytogenetic responses further, irrespective of the need for a third-line treatment, the group adopted the concept of "current CCyR survival" (c-CCyRS), defined as the probability of being alive and in CCyR at a given time point. This essentially is the analog of "current leukemia-free survival," which was developed to describe how patients may relapse but regain remission with an alternative therapy. The c-CCyRS at four years was 54.4%. Furthermore, they demonstrated that by assessing *BCR–ABL1* transcript results at three months, one could potentially identify patients destined to fare poorly [those with >10% BCR–ABL1 transcripts on the International scale (IS) relative to baseline; Fig. 7.3].

As discussed earlier, based on current European Group for Blood and Marrow Transplantation (EBMT) experience, it is reasonable to consider an early allogeneic stem cell transplant (SCT) for those patients who are resistant to imatinib and have high-risk disease, by Sokal and/or Hasford risk stratification, and a low-transplant risk, by EBMT criteria (also known as the Gratwohl score), and wish to be transplanted, rather than receiving a second-generation TKI (Table 4.3).

An alternative approach would be to prescribe a second-generation TKI for a defined period and then proceed with an allogeneic SCT if the response is suboptimal. In practice, however, many patients will opt to receive a trial of dasatinib or nilotinib. Efforts to develop predictive and prognostic scores based on factors known prior to commencing either dasatinib or nilotinib are being developed on both sides of the Atlantic, which might make the decision-making process easier, in particular with regard to balancing the risks associated with an allograft against the risk for disease progression. Clearly, if the notion of the three-month *BCR–ABL1* transcripts is confirmed in larger studies, one could use these results to identify

1. Increase dose of imatinib (600 mg or 800 mg daily)
2. Switch to a second generation TKI (dasatinib or nilotinib)
3. Allogeneic stem cell transplantation (conventional or RIC)
4. Clinical trial

Figure 6.1
Potential treatment options for a patient with chronic myeloid leukemia who has failed imatinib therapy.

patients who should be considered for an alternative therapy. It is of some interest that the NCCN CML 2013 guidelines already feature this milestone analysis, although the evidence is still preliminary. The potential treatment options for patients who are imatinib failures are depicted in Figure 6.1.

A POTENTIAL TREATMENT ALGORITHM FOR A PATIENT WITH CML IN CHRONIC PHASE WHO IS RESISTANT OR INTOLERANT TO ALL CURRENTLY AVAILABLE TKIs

For patients who are resistant/refractory to all of the currently available TKIs and are younger than 50 years, it is probably best to consider an allogeneic SCT, provided that a suitable donor is identified, the patient remains in chronic phase and, of course, wishes to be considered for an allogeneic SCT. It is of note that three candidate drugs, two third-generation TKIs, ponatinib and rebastinib (chapter 1), and a cetaxine, omacetaxine mepesuccinate, are now in clinical trials for patients who are either resistant or intolerant to the second-generation TKIs, and the preliminary results are encouraging for patients who are refractory to multiple TKIs and also those who harbor the T315I subclone. This is discussed in chapter 7. Bosutinib was licensed in September 2012 and ponatinib in December 2012, in USA, for CML patients in chronic phase who have failed a prior TKI; ponatinib was also licensed for all CML patients with a T315I mutation.

For patients who proceed to an allogeneic SCT after prior treatment with TKIs, there is some concern that there might be a higher

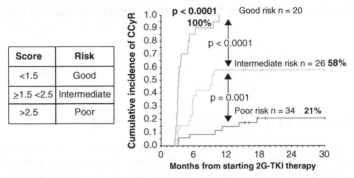

Score	Risk
<1.5	Good
≥1.5 <2.5	Intermediate
>2.5	Poor

Figure 6.2
Hammersmith Hospital Score for predicting CCyR to second-generation TKIs.
Abbreviations: CCyR, complete cytogenetic response; TKIs, tyrosine kinase inhibitors.
Source: From Milojkovic D, Nicholson E, Apperley JF, et al. Early prediction of success
or failure of treatment with second-generation tyrosine kinase inhibitors in patients with
chronic myeloid leukemia. Haematologica 2010; 95: 224–31. A color version of this
figure can be found in Plate VII between pages 46 and 47.

relapse incidence than those who have not previously received TKI. This most likely represents a selection bias for relatively resistant disease. Preliminary data based on small patient series who had previously received imatinib, but not dasatinib or nilotinib, do not, however, suggest that prior treatment with a TKI increases the probability of transplant-related mortality.

Moreover, patients with KD mutations appear to fare as well post-transplant as those lacking such mutations. This is at variance with the current MDACC experience (see above), which suggests that patients with mutations were more likely to develop advanced disease and had worse outcomes after allogeneic SCT. They therefore recommended that allogeneic SCT should be considered early for patients who are considered to have a low probability of responding to a second or subsequent TKI. Efforts are being directed toward the development of predictive and prognostic tools, which could help in this decision-making process. One such effort developed at the Hammersmith Hospital (London) divides patients into three potential risk groups, based on three principal variables: their cytogenetic response to imatinib, the Sokal index at diagnosis, and the occurrence of neutropenia during imatinib treatment (Fig. 6.2).

Another effort from the MDACC group is based on just two variables: the cytogenetic response to imatinib and the performance status at the start of secondary therapy. The notion of screening for *EVI-1* expression at the time of imatinib failure and several biomarkers as a potential predictive marker for response to second-line TKI therapy has also been proposed.

ALLOGENEIC STEM CELL TRANSPLANT

It is remarkable that allogeneic SCT has now been used to treat patients with CML for over three decades. This was the treatment of choice in the pre-imatinib era and in the late 1990s was the most frequent indication for an allogeneic SCT globally. Until 2010, there were conflicting data on a possible adverse effect of prior use of imatinib and there is very little information on children. There is now reasonable evidence that prior imatinib therapy does not alter the outcome of a transplant, but the concerns of a delayed transplant remain. There is also some evidence, at least based on imatinib therapy, that the drug might be less efficacious for adult patients who are classified as "poor-risk" by the Sokal index and consequently some experts had considered offering an allogeneic SCT to these patients, particularly if they were "good-risk" by the EBMT risk stratification score. Many experts also consider transplantation as the preferred primary treatment for children, provided that they have a suitable donor and indeed wish to be transplanted following an informed discussion. Transplantation is also considered for those who either fail to respond to TKI therapy or lose their response thereafter. A topical research approach now is the notion of combining TKI with transplantation. This is attractive since the results of allogeneic SCT for patients in CML who remain in chronic phase show a significant improvement in survival compared with previous decades (Fig. 6.3).

Younger patients, aged 55 years or below, with suitable stem cell donors who fail treatment with TKI may be offered the option of treatment by allogeneic SCT. The major factors influencing survival are patient age, disease phase at the time of SCT, disease duration, degree of histocompatibility between donors and recipients, and gender of donor. In general, patients are "conditioned" for a myeloablative (conventional) transplant with cyclophosphamide at high dosage followed by total body irradiation or with the

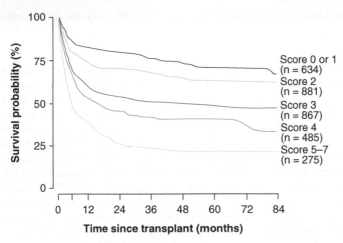

Figure 6.3

Improvements in survival rates by decades of transplantation for patients with CML in chronic phase (courtesy of EBMT registry). Abbreviations: CML, chronic myeloid leukemia; EBMT, European Group for Blood and Marrow Transplantation.

combination of busulfan and cyclophosphamide at high dosage. Reasonable marrow function is typically achieved in three to four weeks after the infusion of donor hematopoietic stem cells.

The possible major complications include graft-versus-host disease (GvHD), reactivation of infection with cytomegalovirus or other viruses, idiopathic pneumonitis, and veno-occlusive disease of the liver. For patients with CML treated by SCT with marrow from HLA-identical siblings, the overall leukemia-free survival (LFS) at five years has steadily improved and is now 60–80%; patients with the lowest EBMT score fare best.

There is a roughly 20% chance of transplant-related mortality and a 15% chance of relapse. Patients surviving without hematological evidence of disease can be monitored by serial cytogenetic studies and by the use of the much more sensitive RQ-PCR, which can detect very low numbers of *BCR–ABL1* transcripts in the blood or marrow. These studies suggest that in the majority of long-term survivors, the CML may truly have been eradicated.

The recognition that the graft versus leukemia (GvL) effect plays a major role in eradicating CML after allografting led to the concept that the toxicity of the transplant procedure could be substantially reduced by decreasing the intensity of the pretransplant conditioning. The resulting strategy is thus to focus predominantly on the use of immunosuppressive rather than myeloablative agents, to maximize the numbers of hematopoietic stem cells transfused, and to exploit the GvL effect mediated by donor alloreactive immunocompetent cells to eliminate the leukemia cells. Procedures such as nonmyeloablative SCTs have been termed variously as reduced-intensity conditioning (RIC) SCTs or mini-SCTs and reflect advances in our understanding of how SCT actually works. It is still too early to say whether such RIC SCTs will prove superior to conventional transplants in the longer term for the younger patient, but the technique could make SCT more widely available to patients at a higher risk and perhaps also to older patients.

The qualified success of conventional SCTs using matched siblings led in the late 1980s to increasing use of "matched" unrelated donors for SCT for patients with CML. At present, unrelated donors matched at low-resolution molecular methods for 6 or 8 HLA antigens can be identified for about 50% of white patients and for lower percentages of patients of other ethnic origins. However, high-resolution molecular methods are now used widely and complete matches for a given patient for 10 gene pairs, HLA-A, -B, -C, -DR, and -DQ, are relatively rare. Thus, in the absence of a "perfect match," the clinician has to decide what degree of mismatch may be acceptable for a given transplant. In general, the results of transplants using such unrelated donors are still somewhat less good than results of using genetically HLA-identical siblings, but some patients can still be cured.

About 10–30% of patients submitted to allogeneic SCT relapse within the first three years post-transplant. The relapse is usually insidious and characterized first by rising levels of *BCR–ABL1* transcripts, then by increasing number of Ph-positive marrow metaphases and, finally (if untreated), by hematological features of chronic-phase disease. This provides some rationale for the recommendation that patients should be monitored post-transplant by regular RQ-PCR and cytogenetic studies. Rare patients in cytogenetic remission relapse directly to advanced-phase disease without any identified intervening period of chronic-phase disease.

For patients with CML in chronic phase treated by allogeneic SCT with marrow from HLA-identical siblings or a matched unrelated donor, the overall LFS at five years is now 80% and 60%, respectively. The transplant-related mortality is about 20% and the chance of relapse is about 15%. Most, but not all, patients who are negative for *BCR–ABL1* transcripts at five years following the allogeneic SCT remain negative for long periods and will probably never relapse (Fig. 4.3).

About 10–30% of patients submitted to allogeneic SCT relapse within the first three years post-transplant. Rare patients in cytogenetic remission relapse directly to advanced-phase disease without any identified intervening period of chronic-phase disease. There are various options for the management of relapse to chronic-phase disease, including use of imatinib, IFN-α, a second transplant using the same or another donor or infusion of lymphocytes from the original donor. Such donor lymphocyte infusions (DLIs) reflect the capacity of lymphoid cells collected from the original transplant donor to mediate a GvL effect although they may have failed to eradicate the leukemia at the time of the original transplant. Recent results of allogeneic SCT reported from the German group who analyzed the results of patients with imatinib-resistant CML in both chronic and advanced phases are encouraging.

TREATMENT FOR RELAPSE OF CML POSTALLOGENEIC STEM CELL TRANSPLANT

In the 10–20% of patients who relapse post-allogeneic SCT for CML, this occurs in the first 3 years. This relapse tends to follow an orderly progression with the patient initially demonstrating evidence of a molecular relapse with increasing positivity of

BCR–ABL1 transcripts by PCR, followed by a cytogenetic relapse when the Ph chromosome is found and then hematological and clinical relapse. Molecular monitoring of all SCT recipients is therefore valuable. For patients with molecular relapse, remission can be re-induced simply by withdrawal of immunosuppression or by the transfusion of donor lymphocytes, providing additional evidence of the potent role of GvL in CML. DLIs can induce remissions in 60–80% of patients with molecular or cytogenetic relapse. The potential benefit of adding TKI to DLI is currently being assessed. Patients who fail to enter remission with DLI may be candidates for a second allogeneic SCT, but the risk of transplant-related mortality is relatively high. Importantly, efforts are also being directed to assess maintenance therapy following allogeneic SCT for imatinib failures, with a second-generation TKI. IFN-α, and other agents, such as 5-azacytidine and other cytotoxic drugs.

CONCLUSIONS

It is of considerable interest to witness how rapidly the potential therapeutic algorithms for patients with CML who do not fare well on first-line therapy, have evolved. The clinical availability of the second-generation TKIs have improved much in terms of both efficacy and safety. The improvements in allogeneic SCT technology over the past decade have accorded this modality to even more prospective candidates and significant gains appear to have been made in the reduction of transplant-associated mortality and morbidity. Importantly, transplantation currently remains the only potential "curative" treatment option for all patients with CML, but particularly so for those in the advanced phase, or harbor a T315I mutation. Table 6.1 depicts the potential indications for an allogeneic SCT today.

Finally, the lessons from transplantation have been instructive in a renewed interest in immunotherapy, and the use of TKIs in conjunction with various immunotherapeutic strategies is now being studied. Parenthetically, it should be noted that globally, so far, our efforts to optimize the clinical management of the newly diagnosed patient have failed. Current estimates, presented by

Table 6.1
Potential Indications for an Allogeneic SCT in CML in 2013

First Chronic Phase
- Failure of second-generation TKI
- Imatinib failure and T315I mutation

Accelerated phase
- Treat like blast crisis if near blast crisis or if enters accelerated phase while on TKI, otherwise as chronic phase

Blast crisis
- Urgently once chronic phase is reestablished with TKI or chemotherapy; consider second-generation TKI postallograft (maintenance)

Abbreviations: CML, chronic myeloid leukemia; SCT, stem cell transplant; TKI, tyrosine kinase inhibitor.

Pasquini and colleagues at the ASH 2011 meeting, suggest that although 81.1% of all patients receive imatinib therapy at some time, most patients are not monitored satisfactorily and therefore have suboptimal outcomes. For some of these patients, it remains reasonable to offer an allogeneic SCT sooner rather than later, as discussed earlier.

7 Emerging and investigational treatment for chronic myeloid leukemia

Despite the notion that the expected survival for most, but not all, patients with chronic myeloid leukemia (CML) now approaches that of the general population, much depends on achieving an optimal response and of course monitoring the patients for response and adverse events appropriately. It is therefore important to continue our efforts in offering patients access to good practice clinical trials that address the issues of optimizing care and potential long-term remissions and probable cure, with the possibility to discontinue the treatments safely. In this chapter, recent efforts in immunotherapy and some of the novel drugs, such as ponatinib, which might offer the potential to improve upon the second-generation tyrosine kinase inhibitors (TKIs), in terms of both efficacy and safety are discussed.

PONATINIB

Ponatinib (formerly called AP24534, Ariad Pharmaceuticals, Cambridge, Massachusetts, USA) is a rationally designed oral inhibitor of *BCR–ABL1* that binds both active and inactive conformations of the enzyme and is active against a broad array of *BCR–ABL1* mutants, including T315I. It has an interesting chemical structure based on a purine scaffold and a central triple carbon-carbon bond with a substructure that is similar to imatinib. The drug inhibits ABL, SRC and a variety of other kinases. Results from the phase I study of this agent, presented in December 2010, which included 32 evaluable patients with CML in chronic phase, demonstrated that 30 (94%) had complete hematologic response (CHR), and 20 (63%) had major cytogenetic response (MCyR): 12 CCyR and eight partial CyR. Remarkably, of 20 CML-chronic-phase cytogenetic responders, 18 remain on treatment [mean duration 326 (range 142–599) days] without progression. There were 11 CML-chronic-phase patients with T315I mutation, 11 (100%) had complete hematologic response (CHR), nine (82%) had MCyR (eight CCyR). Ponatinib may cause pancreatitis in a small proportion of patients, but, overall, it appears to have an acceptable safety profile at therapeutic dose levels and phase III studies are ongoing.

The results of the pivotal phase II trial, Ponatinib Ph-positive ALL and CML Evaluation (PACE), in which 449 patients who were either resistant or intolerant to dasatinib or nilotinib or had a T315I mutation were enrolled, were presented in June 2012 (Table 7.1). The primary endpoint of this trial was an McyR in patients with chronic phase, a major hematological response in patients with the more advanced phases of CML and Ph-positive ALL. The median age was 59 years (range 18–94 years); 53% of all patients were males. In total, at the time the study accrual was closed in September 2011, there were 271 patients in chronic phase, 79 patients in the accelerated phase, and 94 patients either in blast phase or with Ph-positive ALL.

Table 7.1
Responses to Ponatinib Among Patients in the PACE Trial

	n Response to Ponatinib/N Evaluable (%)		
	Overall	R/I	T315I
CP-CML			
MCyR	126/258 (49)	88/197 (45)	38/61 (62)
CCyR	105/258 (41)	70/197 (36)	35/61 (57)
MMR	68/265 (26)	40/205 (20)	28/60 (47)
AP-CML			
MHR	38/57 (67)	31/43 (72)	7/14 (50)
MCyR	27/72 (38)	18/55 (33)	9/17 (53)
CCyR	12/72 (17)	8/55 (15)	4/17 (24)
BC-CML/Ph+ALL			
MHR	33/89 (37)	17/46 (37)	16/43 (37)
MCyR	30/82 (37)	14/41 (34)	16/41 (39)
CCyR	23/82 (28)	11/41 (27)	12/41 (29)

Abbreviations: CCyR, complete cytogenetic response; CML, chronic myeloid leukemia; MCyR, major cytogenetic response; MHR, major hematological response; AP, accelerated phase; BC, blast crisis; CP, chronic phase.
Source: Adapted from Dr Jorge Cortes; table based on data presented at the ASCO meeting, Chicago, June 2012.

Among the chronic-phase patients, 207 were either resistant or intolerant to dasatinib or nilotinib and 64 patients had a T315I mutation; 79 of the accelerated patients and 94 of those in blast phase or Ph-positive ALL were either resistant or intolerant to dasatinib or nilotinib and 19 and 46 had a T315I mutation, respectively. Median time from diagnosis to receiving ponatinib was six years. Prior TKI therapy included imatinib (96%), dasatinib (85%), nilotinib (66%), bosutinib (7%); 94% failed ≥2 prior TKIs, 59% failed ≥3 prior TKIs. Among the patients who were either resistant or intolerant to dasatinib or nilotinib, 83% were resistant and 12% were intolerant. The frequencies of the various kinase domain mutations confirmed at entry into the study were as follows: 29% T315I, 8% F317L, 4% E255K, 4% F359V, and 3% G250E. The median follow-up was 6.6 months.

Forty-seven percent of all patients in chronic phase were able to achieve the primary endpoint of an MCyR. Thrity-nine percent of these patients achieved a CCyR, 33% from resistant/intolerant to dasatinib or nilotinib group and 58% from the T315I cohort; the corresponding MMR results were 19%, 15% and 33%, respectively. At the time of the latest analysis (January 2012), 64% remained on therapy (77% of whom were in chronic phase). The most frequent reasons for discontinuation of ponatinib were disease progression (12%) and side effects (10%). The toxicity data from this PACE trial confirmed thrombocytopenia (33%), rash (33%), and dry skin (26%) to be the most common side effects; Grade 3 (or more) pancreatitis was noted in 6% of the study cohort. Clearly, although longer follow-up is required to establish the precise place of ponatinib in the management of patients with CML who are intolerant or resistant to dasatinib or nilotinib, the data thus far are indeed impressive and confirm the substantial activity of ponatinib in heavily pretreated patients in the various phases of CML and also Ph-positive ALL. Furthermore, it is of note that response rates continue to improve with longer follow-up.

Ponatinib was licensed in December 2012 in the USA for use in adult patients with CML in all phases and also Ph-positive ALL, who have failed prior TKI therapy. The drug's place in the management of those with a T315I mutation is also accepted. It is of interest that the drug was licensed with a 'black box' warning for arterial thrombosis and hepatotoxicity. Ponatinib is now in a phase III trial assessing its candidacy as first-line therapy, compared to imatinib. It may also be useful in treating advanced-phase disease, an area which remains a major treatment challenge. These developments highlight the pace of clinical advancements for our patients with CML and the unprecedented choices for therapy for individual patients.

BOSUTINIB

Bosutinib (formerly SKI-606; Pfizer, New York, New York, USA) an oral dual ABL and SRC kinase inhibitor, is chemically different from both dasatinib and nilotinib. Following single-arm, open-label, multicenter studies assessing bosutinib's role in the treatment of patients with CML in all phases intolerant or resistant/refractory to at least one pior TKI (imatinib), the drug received regulatory approval in the USA in September 2012. It was approved for the treatment of adult patients with chronic- or advanced-phase CML who were resistant or intolerant to prior therapy.

The study cohort comprised 546 patients with CML, of whom 374 patients in the chronic phase and 129 patients in the advanced phases were considered eligible for efficacy analysis: 266 of these patients received prior treatment with only imatinib and 108 patients received prior treatment with imatinib followed by either dastinibor nilotinib. The efficacy endpoints for patients in the chronic phase were the rate and duration of MCyR at week 24, and for patients in the advanced phases were the rate of confirmed CHR and overall hematological response by week 48. In patients with chronic-phase disease who received prior therapy with either one or more than one TKI, 90 [33.8% (95% CI: 28.2, 39.9)] and 29 [26.9% (95% CI: 18.8, 36.2)] achieved MCyR by week 24, respectively. Complete hematological, but not cytogenetic, responses were also seen in about a third of the patients with advanced disease who had had a prior TKI therapy.

It was of note that for the chronic-phase patients who had been treated with prior imatinib only, 53.4% achieved a MCyR at any time during the study; in 52.8% of these, this response lasted at least 18 months. The most common adverse events were diarrhea, nausea, thrombocytopenia, vomiting, abdominal pain, rash, anemia, pyrexia, and fatigue; grade 3/4 adverse events included diarrhea, anaphylactic shock, myelosuppression, fluid retention, hepatoxicity, and rash.

In 2006, bosutinib entered an international randomized, phase III, open-label study of bosutinib versus standard dose imatinib in newly diagnosed patients with CML in chronic phase, called **Bosu**tinib **E**fficacy and Safety in Chronic Myeloid **L**eukemia Study (BELA). A total of 502 newly diagnosed patients with CML in chronic phase were accrued. An intent-to-treat analysis showed that at 12 months, the cumulative rates of CCyR, the primary endpoint of the trial, for bosutinib-treated patients was 70%, compared with 68% for imatinib. The drug therefore failed to meet the US regulatory landmarks to be considered for the first-line approval.

Following a minimum follow-up of 24 months, the cumulative rates of CCyR and MMR in the BELA trial were 87% with bosutinib versus 81% with imatinib, and 67% with bosutinib versus 52% with imatinib, respectively ($P = 0.002$). It is of interest that a lower treatment failure rate was observed in bosutinib-treated patients (4%) compared with those treated with imatinib (13%); additionally, there were fewer progression events on bosutinib (2%) versus imatinib (5%). Bosutinib was associated with higher incidences of gastrointestinal toxicities, in particular grade 3/4 diarrhea, which was noted in 12% of patients. Grade 3/4 liver function abnormalities were also more common in the bosutinib-arm compared with imatinib (23% vs. 4% alanine aminotransferase increase, 12% vs. 4% aspartate aminotransferase increase). Interestingly, the incidence of grade 3/4 neutropenia was less frequent with bosutinib compared to imatinib (11% vs. 24%). These later results of improved molecular response and protection from progression lend some support for the drug's future candidacy for regulatory approval as a first-line therapy.

REBASTINIB

Rebastinib (formerly called DCC-2036, Deciphera Pharmaceuticals, Kansas City, Kansas, USA) is a novel and potent TKI, which binds to a novel region called the switch pocket, thereby preventing

BCR–ABL1 from adopting a conformationally active state. Efficacy against multiple imatinib-resistant BCR–ABL1 mutants has been demonstrated both in vitro and in vivo. Importantly, DCC-2036 retains full potency against the T315I mutant in preclinical efficacy studies. The drug is currently in a phase I study designed to find the maximum tolerated dose (MTD) when administered daily as a single agent on a 28-day cycle. Two reversible dose-limiting toxicities (Grade 3 peripheral neuropathy and Grade 4 lower extremity weakness) occurred during the initial treatment cycle at the 200 mg tablets twice daily dose level. Evaluation of six patients at the 150 mg tablets twice daily dose level determined that dose to be the MTD.

The preliminary results presented in December 2011 from 30 patients with CML in various phases, including 11 patients with the T315I mutation. These preliminary results suggest that rebastinib is well tolerated and has antileukemia activity in subjects with refractory CML and T315I-positive disease. Pharmacokinetics results are consistent with inhibition of *BCR–ABL1* signaling in this first-in-man study of a switch pocket TKI.

OMACETAXINE MEPESUCCINATE

Omacetaxine mepesuccinate (formerly homoharringtonine, Teva-Cephalon, Frazier, Pennyslvania, USA) is a first-in-class cetaxine, which has been in clinical trials for almost two decades, in patients with a variety of hematological malignancies, including CML in various phases. The drug is a natural plant alkaloid from the Chinese plum yew tree, *Cephalotaxus fortunei*, which inhibits synthesis of the antiapoptotic Bcl-2 proteins, and is a potent myelosuppressive agent. It appears to be a reversible, transient inhibitor of protein elongation that facilitates tumor cell death without depending on BCR–ABL1 signaling. Studies in the 1990s confirmed a modest activity in patients with CML, but there were concerns with regard to the route of administration and schedule of delivery largely due to the occurrence of cardiovascular side effects, such as hypotension and arrhythmias. More recently, it has been tested, in a subcutaneously administered formulation, in CML patients resistant to all current TKIs and those who harbor the T315I mutation.

Preliminary results from an MDACC study of 81 patients with CML in various phases confirmed the drugs efficacy and safety in 2010. The best responses were for the patients in chronic phase, with 18% achieving CCyR, following a twice daily subcutaneous administration of the drug. The most frequent nonhematological side effects were diarrhea and headaches. Further phase II studies since have confirmed the drug's clinical activity in "conventional treatment"-resistant patients with different phases of CML.

The results from one of these studies in which 122 such patients resistant/intolerant to ≥2 approved TKIs, were presented in June 2012. Sixty-two of these patients had received two prior TKIs (100% imatinib; 76% dasatinib; 24% nilotinib) and 60 had received all three TKIs. In the 45 patients who had received at least two prior TKIs but remained in chronic phase, there were 12 (27%) MCyRs (median duration of 17.7 months); in the 36 chronic-phase patients subjected to all three TKIs, there were four (11%) MCyRs (median duration not reached). Of the 17 patients in the advanced phases, there were 35% major hematological responses in the two prior TKIs cohort and in the 24 patients who had received three prior TKIs, 21% had major hematological responses. Treatment-related grade 3/4 adverse events were noted in 52 (84%) patients in the two prior TKI group and 42 (70%) in the three prior TKI group; the most common reported side-effect was thrombocytopenia, 71% and 48%, respectively.

Based on these encouraging results in heavily pretreated patients with CML, further studies are ongoing. Should longer follow-up confirm the durability of the responses noted so far, the drug should be a candidate as a salvage agent.

IMMUNOTHERAPY

Following the realization that a complete molecular response (CMR) and "cure" might not be possible with TKI therapy alone, efforts were directed to exploring the potential of developing an active specific immunotherapy strategy for patients with CML by inducing an immune response to a tumor-specific antigen. Furthermore, the demonstration of a powerful graft-versus-leukemia (GvL) effect in CML has renewed interest in the possibility that some form of immunotherapeutic manipulation could be effective in CML. Some evidence suggests that patients vaccinated with oligopeptides corresponding to the junctional region of the BCR–ABL1 protein generate immune responses that may be of clinical benefit.

The principle of immunotherapy in CML involves generating an immune response to the unique amino acid sequence of p210 at the fusion point. Clinical responses to the BCR–ABL1 peptide vaccination, including CCyRs, have been reported in a small series. In contrast to previous earlier unsuccessful attempts, the current series included administration of granulocyte-macrophage colony-stimulating factor (GM-CSF) as an immune adjuvant, and patients were only enrolled if they had measurable residual disease and human leukocyte antigen alleles to which the selected fusion peptides were predicted to bind avidly. If these results can be confirmed, vaccine development against BCR–ABL1 and other CML-specific antigens could become an attractive treatment for patients who have achieved a minimal residual disease status with imatinib.

Other targets for vaccine therapy now being studied include peptides derived from the Wilms tumor-1 (WT-1) protein, proteinase-3 (PR1), PRAME, and elastase, all of which are overexpressed in CML cells. Another vaccine strategy that may prove useful for patients who do not achieve a CCyR to imatinib is use of the K562 CML cell line engineered to produce GM-CSF.

CONCLUSION

The late 2012 licensing of bosutinib and ponatinib for patients with CML who have failed prior TKI should be considered another major step in the CML treatment success story. The candidacy of both these drug's as potential first-line therapy is now being tested against imatinib. Immunotherapy is also garnering support, in particular with the BCR–ABL1 and other CML-specific antigens' targeted vaccines for patients following TKI-induced minimal residual disease status.

It is also of note that most current CML clinical trials have focused on the effects of a specific drug (monotherapy) rather than a specific treatment strategy. This is even more important when the salvage therapies are quite effective and able to promote responses in a significant majority of patients who fail or are intolerant to the initial drug therapy. This is highlighted by the recent success of drugs, such as ponatinib, which are indicative of the necessity to design future clinical trials that focus on specific treatment strategies.

8 Definitions of response and monitoring response for patients with chronic myeloid leukemia

INTRODUCTION

A decade following the introduction of the original tyrosine kinase inhibitor (TKI), imatinib, into the clinics for the treatment of patients with chronic myeloid leukemia (CML) in chronic phase, it is abundantly clear that the overall safety and efficacy of the drug are impressive but not optimal. It induces complete cytogenetic response (CCyR) rates of 65–85%, major molecular response (MMR; defined as a 3-log or more reduction in the *BCR–ABL1* transcript levels compared with the baseline) rates of 40–70%, and a complete molecular response (CMR; defined as the absence of any detectable *BCR–ABL1* transcripts) rates of 10–40%.

Imatinib is not optimal treatment because it appears to improve the outcomes for only about 60% of patients. In the quest to improve upon these treatment results, the necessity to improve monitoring of minimal residual disease (MRD) was recognized. Over the past several years we have witnessed the development of the next generation of TKIs, which are more potent in their activity in CML compared with imatinib. We have also witnessed important changes in monitoring of CML patients on TKI therapy and of being able to "quantify" the degree of disease burden better. At the inception of the IRIS trial, response was expressed in three separate, but integrated parameters: hematological, cytogenetic, and molecular response (Table 8.1).

Hematological responses are defined as the normalization of peripheral blood counts, absence of immature cells from the blood, and normalization of the spleen size. Cytogenetic responses, using

Table 8.1
Definitions of Response in Chronic Myeloid Leukemia

Response by Type	Definitions
Hematologic	
Complete (CHR)	WBC < 10 × 10⁹/L
	Basophils < 5%
	No myelocytes, promyelocytes, myeloblasts in the differential
	Platelet count < 450 × 10⁹/L
	Spleen nonpalpable
Cytogenetic*	
Complete (CCyR)	No Ph + metaphases
Partial (PCgR)	1% to 35% Ph + metaphases
Minor (mCgR)	36% to 65% Ph + metaphases
Minimal (mkinCgR)	66% to 95% Ph + metaphases
None (noCgR)	>95% Ph + metaphases
Molecular†	
Complete (CMolR)	Undetectable *BCR–ABL* mRNA transcripts by real-time quantitative and/or nested PCR in two consecutive blood samples of adequate quality (sensitivity > 10⁴)
Major (MMolR)	Ratio of *BCR–ABL* to *ABL* (or other housekeeping genes) ≤ 0.1% on the international scale

Abbreviation: CHR, complete hematoloigc response.

conventional karyotyping techniques, are defined as complete (CCyR) (undetectable Ph-positive cells), partial (PCyR) (1–35% Ph-positive cells in bone marrow metaphase), minor (mCyR) (>95% Ph-positive cells), and major cytogenetic response (MCyR) (includes CCyR and PCyR). These definitions were established based on the association of MCyR and CCyR with improved long-term survival during the IFN-α era; the prognostic association was thereafter confirmed with imatinib therapy and the notion that response and survival may actually be independent of the treatment that resulted in a response. Molecular responses are defined by real-time quantitative polymerase chain reaction (RT-qPCR) procedures that quantify the *BCR–ABL1* transcript copy numbers. Molecular responses are defined as MMR (of at least 3-log reduction in the *BCR–ABL1* transcripts ratio compared with a standardized

Table 8.2
Definitions of Complete Molecular Response

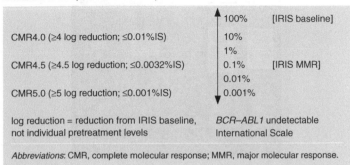

	100%	[IRIS baseline]
CMR4.0 (≥4 log reduction; ≤0.01%IS)	10%	
	1%	
CMR4.5 (≥4.5 log reduction; ≤0.0032%IS)	0.1%	[IRIS MMR]
	0.01%	
CMR5.0 (≥5 log reduction; ≤0.001%IS)	0.001%	
log reduction = reduction from IRIS baseline, not individual pretreatment levels	*BCR–ABL1* undetectable International Scale	

Abbreviations: CMR, complete molecular response; MMR, major molecular response.

baseline obtained from patients with untreated newly diagnosed CML) and CMR (undetectable *BCR–ABL1* transcripts). Currently, there are several slightly different definitions of CMR, clearly with somewhat diverse significances (Table 8.2).

Historically, cytogenetic analysis has been the mainstay of MRD monitoring and considered by many, but not all, experts as the "gold" standard for evaluating response to TKI therapy in patients with CML. It does, however, has several limitations, in particular being rather time consuming and importantly at least 20 metaphases need to be examined in a particular sample. These aspects can sometimes make the estimate of the percentage of Ph-positive cells imprecise. These limitations led to the use of fluorescence in situ hybridization (FISH) that is performed by co-hybridization of BCR and ABL1 probes. This technology and evolved from an "interphase" (i-FISH) to a much more sensitive "hypermetaphase" FISH. FISH analysis cannot detect other chromosomal abnormalities apart from the Ph chromosome (Fig. 8.1). It can be carried out on a peripheral blood sample and can be useful when conventional cytogenetic analysis is unhelpful. Parenthetically it should be noted that studies associating cytogenetic response with long-term prognosis have been based on conventional cytogenetics, and not FISH. Table 8.3 depicts the different methods available in clinical practice to detect residual leukemia.

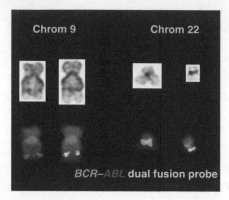

Figure 8.1
A photomicrograph of dual fluorescence in situ hybridization analysis for the BCR–ABL1 fusion gene. A color version of this figure can be found in Plate VIII *between pages 46 and 47.*

Table 8.3
Methods to Detect Residual Leukemia in 2013

Method	Target	Tissue	Sensitivity (%)
Marrow cytogenetics	Ph-chromosome	BM	1–10
FISH	Juxtaposition of BCR and ABL1	PB/BM	0.2–5
Southern blotting	M–BCR rearrangement	PB/BM	1–10
Western blotting	BCR–ABL1 protein	PB/BM	0.2–1
RQ-PCR	BCR–ABL1 mRNA	PB/BM	0.001–0.0001

Abbreviation: FISH, fluorescence in situ hybridization.

Based on the notion that most patients with CML in chronic phase will have a total burden of about 10^{12} Ph-positive cells at diagnosis, and assuming a maximum sensitivity of 1% for conventional cytogenetics and FISH, a patient with negative results may harbor as many as 10^{10} Ph-positive cells; Figure 8.2 depicts the notion of the *BCR–ABL1* amount paralleling the mathematical number of Ph-positive cells.

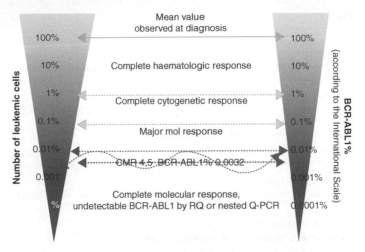

Figure 8.2
The BCR–ABL1 Amount Parallels the Number of Ph-positive cells.

In 1989, when PCR monitoring entered the CML clinical arena, the test was a qualitative test (RT-PCR) that could identify the presence or absence of *BCR–ABL1* transcripts and was useful in monitoring patients with CML subjected to an allogeneic stem cell transplant (SCT). However, it was assumed that patients who were negative by RT-PCR could in their body harbor as many as 10^7 Ph-positive cells! This was therefore replaced by the current RT-qPCR technology.

MONITORING STRATEGIES FOR PATIENTS WITH CML IN CHRONIC PHASE ON TKIs

The principal objective of monitoring patients with CML is to accurately determine response to treatment and be able to detect relapse at an early stage, particularly if a change of treatment might be indicated. Remarkably similar monitoring approaches have been proposed by the European LeukemiaNet (ELN) and many CML-interested consortia (Table 8.4).

Table 8.4

Monitoring Patients who are on Tyrosine Kinase Inhibitor Therapy

Hematologic
- At diagnosis, then every 2 weeks until complete hematologic response, then every 3 months for 2 years, then 3–6 monthly

Cytogenetic (bone marrow)
- At diagnosis, at 3 months, and at 6 months; thereafter every 6 monthly until CCyR confirmed. Once CCyR is confirmed, monitor with FISH or qPCR. Repeat bone marrow if clinically indicated

Molecular by RT-qPCR (peripheral blood)
- RT-qPCR every 3 months until MMR confirmed, then every 6 months

FISH (peripheral blood)
- If unable to perform conventional cytogenetics on bone marrow; or once CCyR confirmed, can be used to supplement qPCR results

Mutational analysis (peripheral blood)
- Only if failure (required before decision to change treatment)

Abbreviations: CCyR, complete cytogenetic response; FISH, fluorescence in situ hybridization; RT-qPCR, real-time quantitative polymerase chain reaction.

Despite these efforts, there appears to be a monitoring paradigm shift, initially in the USA and now global, of using molecular monitoring in preference to cytogenetics (see below). Molecular monitoring is indeed an important aspect of the management of patients with CML, but its principal role, outside of clinical trials, appears to be in the patient who has achieved a firm CCyR. Table 8.5 depicts the revised ELN criteria for responses in patients with CML in chronic phase initially treated with TKIs.

The frequency of performing a specific test has been based largely on the results from the IRIS study and other global single institutions and consortia trials. For example, in patients with CCyR, molecular monitoring with FISH and RQ-PCR is recommended every six months, rather than every three months, based on the IRIS study demonstrating the low risk of transformation to the advanced phases beyond the second year. Most experts appear to prefer peripheral blood analyses for monitoring, rather than bone marrow studies, except at diagnosis. The ELN guidelines require bone marrow conventional cytogenetics at diagnosis, at three and

Table 8.5

Revised European LeukemiaNet (ELN) Criteria for Responses in Patients with Chronic Myeloid Leukemia in Chronic Phase Initially Treated with TKIs

	Response Definition and Criteria from the ELN			
Milestone	Optimal	Suboptimal	Warning	Failure
3 months	CHR + minor CyR	No CyR	N/A	<CHR
6 months	PCyR	<PCyR	N/A	No CyR
12 months	CCyR	PCyR	<MMR	<PCyR
18 months	MMR	<MMR	N/A	<CCyR
Any time	Stable or improving MMR	Loss of MMR, imatinib sensitive mutations	↑ transcript levels, clonal chromosomal abnormalities	Loss of CyR or CHR, imatinib insensitive mutations

Abbreviations: CCyR, complete cytogenetic response; CHR, complete hematologic response; FISH, fluorescence in situ hybridization; MMR, major molecular response; RT-qPCR, real-time quantitative polymerase chain reaction.
Source: From Baccarani M, Cortes J, Pane F, et al. Chronic myeloid leukemia: an update of concepts and management recommendations of European LeukemiaNet. J Clin Oncol 2009; 27: 6041–51.

six months, and then every six months until CCyR has been confirmed. Once a stable CCyR has been achieved, it is reasonable to monitor responses every six months, because abrupt transformation to advanced phases are quite rare. Finally, it is important to monitor compliance throughout the treatment period. Several studies have demonstrated the critical importance of adherence in terms of achieving optimal outcomes.

Baseline Investigation

All CML patients should be assessed thoroughly as any patient, with a detailed history and clinical examination. All patients should then have a complete blood count, blood chemistry (renal, hepatic profile) bone marrow aspirate/biopsy for morphology and conventional cytogenetic analysis, and RQ-PCR on peripheral blood sample. The conventional cytogenetics will confirm the diagnosis, provide information for Sokal index, and also detect clonal evolution (if any). A FISH can detect Ph-negative but *BCR–ABL1*-positive disease. Patients who are commenced on TKI therapy, should be followed regularly for hematological, cytogenetic, and molecular response (Table 8.3).

Hematological Response

Complete hematological response (CHR) is defined as a white blood count (WBC) $<10 \times 10^9$/L with the differential count showing no immature granulocyte, basophils <5%, platelet count $<450 \times 10^9$/L, and no palpable spleen. In the IRIS study, 96% of all patients achieved CHR by 12 months and 98% at 60 months. A failure to achieve CHR by three months is considered as imatinib failure. In the IRIS study some patients develop grade 3–4 cytopenias, in particular neutropenia (17%), thrombocytopenia (9%), and anemia (4%) and might require discontinuing the drug or reducing the dose (preferable). In most patients the cytopenias are short-lived, but some patients with severe neutropenia might require a hematopoietic growth factor, such as G-CSF, support. It is important to maintain the dose intensity of the TKI as best as possible. The ELN guidelines suggest that peripheral blood count should be monitored two weekly until CHR is achieved and then three monthly thereafter unless otherwise required.

Cytogenetic Response

Most experts concur that a baseline bone marrow examination is desirable and conventional cytogenetics could be carried out. The bone marrow examination with conventional cytogenetics should be repeated three monthly until CCyR and then cytogenetics can be monitored solely by FISH analysis, carried out three monthly. Some clinicians prefer not to do bone marrow examinations at all and rather obtain FISH analysis on peripheral blood sample. This is not preferred for the reasons discussed above, but if it is carried out, FISH should be repeated every three months until the FISH levels are less than 5–10%, when a bone marrow evaluation with conventional cytogenetics be done to confirm a CCyR. Thereafter, it is reasonable to monitor the patient with regular FISH studies, provided they are reported as negative; persistent low levels of FISH positivity should trigger a conventional cytogenetic analysis.

The IRIS study established that cytogenetic response at three and six months predicts CCyR and progression-free survival (PFS) at 24 months. Subsequent follow-up of the trial suggested that a cytogenetic response at six months is a better predictor than a cytogenetic response at six months. It is therefore reasonable to perform a bone marrow conventional cytogenetic analysis at baseline, at six months, and then six monthly until the patient achieves a CCyR. Patients who experience a significant rise in the *BCR–ABL1* transcripts levels and loss of their MMR by RQ-PCR, should be considered for a repeat bone marrow conventional cytogenetic examination. If there is evidence of an additional clonal event, then the clinician might contemplate a change of therapy.

Molecular Monitoring

It is desirable, but not mandatory, for all patients to have a baseline RT-qPCR for *BCR–ABL1* on peripheral blood and thereafter three monthly after the confirmation of CCyR. The IRIS trial is considered to have provided evidence that a reduction of the *BCR–ABL1* transcripts was predictive of PFS. In the landmark analysis of the trial, achievement of MMR versus no MMR by 12 months was associated with improved event-free survival (EFS), but not with improved overall survival (OS). A subsequent re-analysis showed that 18 months MMR did correlate with sustained CCyR and OS. Thereafter, many studies have addressed the precise significance of achieving MMR at specific milestones.

In general the importance of achieving MMR has been recognized, but the notion of defining the patients who do not achieve MMR is challenging. These patients represent a rather motley group, including those who are in CCyR but not MMR and some in CHR but neither CCyR nor MMR.

An important predictor of long-term response to TKI therapy is the depth of response at early time points. The Adelaide group have demonstrated that *BCR–ABL1* mRNA levels assessed by PCR after only three months of therapy is strongly associated with achievement of CCyR, MMR, and PFS. Conversely, patients who did not have a 1-log (10-fold) reduction of their *BCR–ABL1* transcripts by three months had a very low probability of achieving MMR (13% at 30 months). Those who achieved a >2-log (100-fold) reduction at three months (this is equivalent to achieving a CCyR, by conventional cytogenetics) had a 100% probability of achieving MMR. More recently studies have addressed the usefulness of cytogenetic and *BCR–ABL1* transcripts results following three months of first-line TKI therapy (Table 8.6).

The efforts reporting the usefulness of the *BCR–ABL1* transcripts at three months as a predictive parameter for patients receiving TKI therapy suggest the critical cutoff point to be at the 10% international scale (IS) level, where patients with a *BCR–ABL1* of >10% IS fared poorly compared with those whose disease burden was <10% (see Table 4.3). These potentially useful parameters need further validation prior to being used in the clinics to identify patients who should be considered for an alternative therapy.

Table 8.6
Three-Month Responses and Outcomes on TKI Therapy

Drug	3 Months Response Level	Outcomes	Abstract
Imatinib	CCyR	EFS 83% vs 35%	3783
Imatinib	*BCR–ABL1* transcripts 10% IS	cCCyR 91% vs 47% OS 93% vs 57%	1680
Imatinib +/– Interferon	*BCR–ABL1* transcripts 10% IS	FFS 94% vs 86% EFS 86% vs 65%	1684
Nilotinib or Dasatinib	*BCR–ABL1* transcripts 10% IS	OS 97% vs 87%	783
Dasatinib	*BCR–ABL1* transcripts 10% IS	CCyR 93% vs 76% MMR 83% vs 54% CMR 20% vs 0%	785

Abbreviations: CCyR, complete cytogenetic response; cCCyR, continuous complete cytogenetic response; MMR, major molecular response; CMR, complete molecular response; EFS, event-free survival; OS, overall survival; FFS, failure-free survival; vs, versus; TKI, tyrosine kinase inhibitors; IS, international scale.

The measurement of *BCR–ABL1* transcripts by RT-PCR is most relevant in patients that have achieved a CCyR. After seven years of follow-up in the IRIS study, no patients achieving CCyR and MMR at 18 months had progressed to advanced phase. The rate of progression for those that had a CCyR but less than 3-log reduction in *BCR–ABL1* was only 3%. Subsequent studies have confirmed the IRIS PCR data and demonstrate that patients with a deeper molecular response at the time of initial CCyR, or a >3-log reduction of *BCR–ABL1* during CCyR, have very low odds of progression and a superior PFS compared with patients with an inferior response.

Despite being the qualified method of choice to monitor patients who have achieved a CCyR, there are several challenges. There appears much diversity in not only how the test is carried out, but also how the results are reported in different laboratories. Many of the methods appear not to have been standardized and there appears to be some variability in the guidelines for acceptable levels of reproducibility and sensitivity of the procedure. In the context of the IRIS trial, the standardized baseline was defined as the average ratio from 30 patients was 36%. An MMR was therefore "defined" as achieving levels of 0.036% or less. The considerable range in the values among the study cohort introduces some uncertainty to the results. Moreover, this standardized baseline required to be stringently applied in individual laboratories, a feat not easily accepted by many commercial laboratories, resulting in significant interlaboratory variations; some laboratories do not even include this baseline in the final report.

A major effort led by John Goldman (London) is to establish a harmonization of results from diverse laboratories in diverse countries began in Bethesda in October 2006 and is currently ongoing. A significant step has been to develop accredited reference reagents that are directly linked to the *BCR–ABL1* international scale, under the aegis of the World Health Organization (WHO; as the WHO International Genetic Reference Panel). Once this has been accomplished, a conversion factor should follow and the individual laboratories can adjust their values uniformly to define MMR as a value of 0.1% or less on the adjusted scale. It is of interest that even in the "best" laboratories there can be a log-0.5 (fivefold) variation in the reported results. Efforts on the use of a DNA-based RT-qPCR, which would be "patient specific" rather than the RNA-based "disease specific," are also ongoing. For the moment, on a lighter note, we remind ourselves of the quotation from William Shakespeare:

> *"Men do their broken weapons rather use/than their bare hands"* (The Doge's advice to Brabantio) Othello, act I, scene 3!

Mutational Analysis

Studies designed to detect acquired mutations in the kinase domain of the *BCR–ABL1* gene are generally not indicated when treatment with TKI therapy is commenced. They are also of very limited value in patients who are responding appropriately on therapy. The studies themselves are costly and not readily available, so it is imperative to perform them when the results should require a change in therapy, unless the patients are in a clinical trial that stipulates the need. The 2011 ELN-led *BCR–ABL1* kinase domain mutation analysis guidelines recommend mutational studies to be performed only with evidence of failure or suboptimal response or if there is a therapy change. The later is particularly important since the choice of the next therapy might well be dictated in part by the demonstration of specific mutations, for example, if the T315I mutation, a preferred treatment might be an allogeneic SCT, or perhaps ponatinib, if the mature analysis confirms its efficacy and safety.

Blood Levels of Imatinib

There has been some interest in monitoring imatinib blood levels to optimize the imatinib dose-intensity. This was based on pharmacokinetic studies of the four-week trough blood level of imatinib and its correlation with cytogenetic and molecular response and suggestions that high blood levels might correlate with some imatinib-related toxicities. Patients who maintained an imatinib trough level >1000 ng/mL were noted to have a greater probability of achieving a CCyR. A Hammersmith Hospital (London) study assessing potential independent prognostic factors for optimal long-term outcome confirmed that imatinib blood level *per se* was not an independent prognostic factor. At present there are no data from randomized studies necessitating a change in imatinib dose based on blood levels and most experts would agree that imatinib blood levels, outside of a clinical trial, are not required. With this regard, the current Australian trial (TIDEL-II), in which patients with CML in chronic phase have imatinib doses increased from 600 to 800 mg daily based on a day 22 imatinib plasma level of <1000 ng/mL should be of interest.

RELEVANT LONG-TERM ENDPOINTS DURING TKI THERAPY IN SOME CHALLENGING ISSUES WITH REGARD TO MONITORING CML PATIENTS

What Should One Do with a Rising BCR–ABL1 PCR?

First, the PCR assessment should be repeated. The *BCR–ABL1* qPCR may rise in a patient for a number of reasons. One possibility relates to compliance, especially in the context of an expensive drug (i.e., any TKI) and a patient with a good molecular response and/or in the presence of chronic insidious side effects (a situation where the temptation to enjoy a "drug holiday" is strong). Secondly, results may "wobble" due to sampling error (especially in the presence of a very low tumor burden), and the intrinsic variability of the test itself. In most laboratories, however, a 5- to 10-fold change in the RT-qPCR is likely "real"; the Oregon CML group recently reported a 2.6-fold rise to correlate with risk of loss of MMR and cytogenetic relapse. However, it is not known how *BCR–ABL1* levels vary in patients naturally over time while on TKI therapy.

The natural history of CML in chronic phase is known to be associated with cyclic oscillations with peaks and troughs occurring at even one- to two-month intervals, and this has not been studied in cases with residual disease. Clearly the most important possible explanation for an increase in *BCR–ABL1* is an impending relapse.

Minor changes in *BCR–ABL1* levels should not trigger any change in therapy. However, loss of MMR, never achieving MMR, or experiencing an increase in *BCR–ABL1* mRNA transcript levels >1-log should be very closely monitored.

What Should One Do for a Patient with CML Who Is in Confirmed CCyR But Not MMR?

A topical current question is the importance of achieving MMR in a patient who is in CCyR, or one who loses his/her MMR but remains in CCyR. This issue has significant practical implications and appears not to be addressed in the latest ELN response and treatment guidelines (but anticipated to be addressed in the late 2013 updates). The ELN takes a stance for patients who have a suboptimal response, but there is some concern with regard to suboptimal responses in general. Many experts feel that it is reasonable to monitor such patients more stringently and perhaps perform a mutational analysis (see below) in those who have lost MMR. At present, there seem to be no studies that have addressed the notion of a change of therapy for patients who have a suboptimal response but are in CCyR. There is, of course, firm data to support such a change of therapy for those who have lost their CCyR.

In a Hammersmith Hospital (London) study, an outcome analysis of 204 patients with newly diagnosed CML in chronic phase treated with standard dose imatinib suggested that those who achieved CCyR by 12 months had significantly better rates of PFS and OS. The achievement of MMR for this cohort appeared not to improve outcome further. A similar MD Ande rson Cancer Center (Houston) study enrolling 276 patients with newly diagnosed CML in chronic phase treated with imatinib revealed a better PFS and OS for those who achieved an MCyR between 6 and 12 months; patients who in addition achieved MMR demonstrated a better PFS, but not OS compared with those in CCyR. Finally, the German CML Study Group published their results of the tolerability-adapted imatinib 800 mg/day versus 400 mg/day versus 400 mg/day plus interferon-α in newly diagnosed CML in April 2011. These investigators noted that achieving MMR in a cohort already in CCyR might not confer additional outcome benefit. Such observations perhaps add to the debate of the optimal early therapeutic endpoints in clinical trials for patients with CML in chronic phase receiving TKI therapy. There is, of course, no doubt that the additional achievement of MMR for the patients in CCyR must reduce subsequent CML-related events, such as transformation to advanced phases, which would be associated with an inferior outcome.

CONCLUSION AND SOME THOUGHTS ON APPROPRIATE LONG-TERM ENDPOINTS IN TKI-BASED CLINICAL TRIALS FOR PATIENTS WITH CML IN CHRONIC PHASE

Just over a decade since the original TKI, imatinib, entered the clinics and literally revolutionized the treatment algorithm for patients with CML, we now have two second-generation TKIs, dasatinib and nilotinib, which are licensed for first-line treatment, and also two potential first-line candidate drugs, bosutinib and ponatinib. Dasatinib and nilotinib have so far fared considerably better than imatinib in randomized studies of first-line treatment for patients with CML in chronic phase, in terms of achieving a higher rate of CCyR and MMR at the landmark analysis carried out following 12 months of therapy. Furthermore, nilotinib appears to alter the natural history of CML, by reducing the risk of transforming into the advanced phases of the disease, compared with imatinib; the progression rate on dasatinib versus imatinib in the DASISION trial has not been statistically significant so far.

One of our biggest challenges appears to be the demonstration of a significant survival benefit for the second-generation TKIs and indeed the next generation of candidate drugs. Imatinib therapy has accorded for patients with CML in chronic phase a survival (OS) of at least 85% at 10 years. To demonstrate statistically significant OS and EFS benefits for the next wave of treatments would clearly require the daunting task of recruiting large numbers of patients into large randomized prospective trials that would require lengthy follow-up at a considerable cost. Moreover, it will be helpful if the future trials could have homogenous definitions of the different endpoints and events.

9 Resistance to tyrosine kinase inhibitors and novel insights into genomic instability of chronic myeloid leukemia stem cells

Defining responses to imatinib and other tyrosine kinase inhibitor (TKI) therapy and monitoring of patients with CML, have been a challenge for some time. Various efforts to define failure and suboptimal responses have resulted in the two principal consensus panels, the European LeukemiaNet (ELN) and the MD Anderson Cancer Center (MDACC) panels, not necessarily mutually exclusive, which focus on achieving well-defined responses at specific time points (see chap. 8); others, such as the National Comprehensive Cancer Network (NCCN) chronic myeloid leukemia (CML) task force in the USA have also complied remarkably similar criteria. The initial goals of therapy are ideally to achieve a complete hematologic response (CHR) by three months and a complete cytogenetic response (CCyR) by 12 months. It is of some interest that slow responders who eventually achieve a CCyR may not necessarily have a significantly worse prognosis than those who achieve this landmark by the "ideal" 12 months period. This provides some rationale for continuing imatinib in patients who have not met the milestones stipulated in some of the current guidelines, such as the ELN, and do not have a useful alternative treatment available. Resistance to TKI therapy in general can be divided into primary and secondary. The issue of resistance is therefore clearly more complex than simply lack or loss of some predefined responses at specific times.

PRIMARY RESISTANCE

Primary resistance or refractoriness to imatinib is very rare and it is likely to reflect underlying heterogeneity of CML at diagnosis. It can be associated with low levels of the human organic cation transporter type 1 (hOCT-1), which are associated with poor intracellular uptake of imatinib, or with a poorly compliant patient (Fig. 9.1).

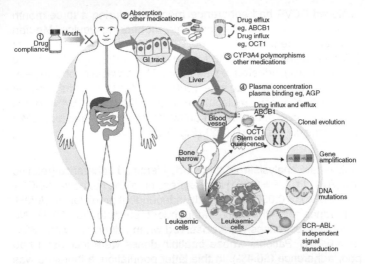

Figure 9.1
Mechanisms of imatinib resistance in patients with CML in chronic phase. Abbreviations: *CML, chronic myeloid leukemia; GI, gastrointestinal.* Source: *Courtesy of Professor Jane Apperley.*

Recent in vitro studies suggest that SHP-1 expression is significantly lower in CML cell lines resistant to imatinib compared with those sensitive to imatinib. The investigators proposed that SHP-1 had the potential to be considered as a predictive marker of imatinib sensitivity at baseline. Other genetic candidates for primary resistance include novel deletion polymorphism in the *BIM* gene. Investigators from Singapore found this abnormality to be present in East-Asians (12.3%), compared with African or Caucasian-populations, and correlated with imatinib resistance both clinically and *in vitro*.

Clearly compliance plays a far bigger role than previously perceived and when seen may be related to poor compliance, abnormal drug efflux and influx, poor gastrointestinal absorption, p450 cytochrome polymorphism, and interactions with other medications. In a Hammersmith Hospital (London) study, 87 patients with CML in chronic phase were treated with imatinib 400 mg/day for a median of 59.7 months (range, 25–104 months) who had achieved CCyR had adherence monitored during a three-month period by using a microelectronic monitoring device. Median adherence rate was 98% (range, 24–104%). Just over one quarter (26.4%) of the patients had adherence ≤90%; in 12 of these patients (14%), adherence was ≤80%. There was a strong correlation between adherence rate (≤90% or >90%) and the six-year probability of a major molecular response (MMR) of 28.4% versus 94.5% for those not achieving an MMR ($P < 0.001$) and also CMR 0% versus 43.8% ($P = 0.002$) (Fig. 9.2).

Multivariate analysis from this study identified adherence [relative risk (RR), 11.7; $P = 0.001$] and expression of the molecular hOCT1 (RR, 1.79; $P = 0.038$) as the only independent predictors for MMR. Adherence was the only independent predictor for CMR. No molecular responses were observed when adherence was ≤80% ($P < 0.001$). Patients whose imatinib doses were increased had poor adherence (86.4%). In this latter population, adherence was the only independent predictor for inability to achieve an MMR

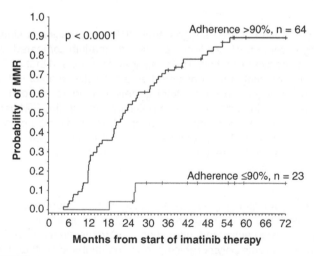

Figure 9.2
A six-year probability of MMR according to adherence rate. Abbreviation: *MMR, major molecular response.* Source: *Courtesy of Professor John Goldman, presented at ASH 2010.*

(RR, 17.66; $P = 0.006$). In a small cohort of patients a correlation of hOCT1 expression and molecular response has been confirmed, with those with the higher levels of hOCT1 demonstrating the best responses. Similar findings have been observed in the Adherence Assessment with Glivec: Indicators and Outcomes (ADAGIO) study.

SECONDARY RESISTANCE

About 30% of patients in chronic phase and almost all of those in blast crisis become resistant to the inhibitory effects of all the TKIs currently in clinical use (imatinib, dasatinib, and nilotinib). It is, of course, quite interesting that, although these powerful drugs eventually eliminate the majority of leukemia progenitor cells (LPCs) in patients responding to the treatment, their effect on leukemia stem cells (LSCs) is considered negligible. Patients with CML in chronic phase harbor approximately 5×10^7 leukemia cells displaying innate resistance to TKIs. These cells may accumulate additional genetic aberrations causing acquired resistance to TKIs and progression to advanced phase. TKI resistance may be induced not only by mutations in the kinase domain of BCR–ABL1, but also by mutations in genes other than BCR–ABL1.

The mechanism for secondary or acquired resistance whereby patients respond well initially and then lose their response, appear quite different. Acquired resistance can conveniently be considered as either BCR–ABL1 *independent* or BCR–ABL1 *dependent* (Fig. 9.3). *BCR–ABL1*-independent resistance may arise if a CML cell acquires additional molecular changes that cannot be targeted by imatinib. Thus far, there is little known about such events.

Conversely *BCR–ABL1*-dependent resistance may be due to changes that specifically involve the BCR–ABL1 oncoprotein. The principal mechanism underlying this form of resistance appears to involve expansion of a Ph-positive clone bearing a *BCR–ABL1* kinase domain (KD) mutation. It can also arise from a variety of other mechanisms, including amplification of the *BCR–ABL1* fusion gene, relative overexpression of BCR–ABL1 oncoprotein or overexpression of the *MDR-1* gene and encoded P-glycoprotein that could lead to excessive expulsion of the inhibitor from the cell.

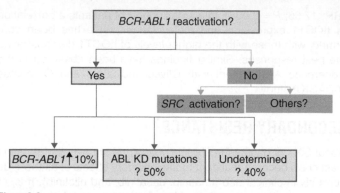

Figure 9.3
Mechanisms of acquired resistance to imatinib.

In 2012, Talpaz and Donato, in Michigan, have reported on activation of *SRC* family kinases in acquired imatinib resistance.

Currently over 80 different mutations in the ABL1 kinase domain have been identified in association with acquired resistance to imatinib; mutations that result in structural changes, which prevent imatinib binding but do not prevent pathological phosphorylation of the relevant substrates by the oncoprotein, tend to be multiple and confer polyclonal resistance to imatinib.

Such mutations probably reflect selection by imatinib of mutations already present at a low level before initiation of treatment rather than *de novo* acquisition during imatinib therapy. Since the reactivation of the inappropriate *BCR–ABL1* signaling is a principal finding in CML cells, which develop resistance to imatinib, efforts have focused on the efforts to re-establish ABL1 tyrosine kinase inhibition. Dose escalation of imatinib overcomes clinical resistance in some but not all patients, and response appears to depend on the specific mutation. There is some evidence to suggest that the mutational analysis could be used to select the type of alternative therapy (Table 9.1).

A somewhat larger proportion of patients, about 20% in the chronic phase, responds initially to imatinib and then loses their response.

Table 9.1
Mutational Analysis and Potential Selection of Next-Line Therapy

T315I
• Consider allogeneic SCT or ponatinib or an investigational drug
V299L, T315A, F315L/V/I/C
• Consider nilotinib rather than dasatinib
Y253H, E255K, E255V, F359V/C/I
• Consider dasatinib rather than nilotinib
Abbreviation: SCT, stem cell transplant.

Some of these patients show evidence of expansion of subclones with point mutations in the BCR–ABL1 KD, which code for amino acid substitutions that may impede binding of imatinib but do not impair phosphorylation of downstream substrates that mediate the leukemia signal. The precise position of the mutation appears to dictate the degree of resistance to imatinib; some mutations are associated with minor degrees of imatinib resistance, whereas one notorious mutation, the replacement of threonine by isoleucine at position 315 (T315I), is associated with near total nonresponsiveness to imatinib as well as with resistance to the second-generation TKIs. The precise significance and indeed the kinetics of the various mutations remain largely unelucidated.

Structural studies suggest that not all mutations are equivalent; T315I and some (but not all) P-loop mutations, such as E255K, are associated with resistance to imatinib, probably because they interfere with imatinib-binding to the BCR–ABL1 KD. Currently there is debate about the significance of these mutations in CML, particularly since some mutations have been identified at a very low level in newly diagnosed patients and probably reflect the natural evolution of the CML stem cells. It is however becoming increasingly clearer that patients with multiple low-level mutations fare poorly with second-line TKI therapies (Table 9.2).

Cells harboring TKI-resistant BCR–ABL1 kinase mutants appear to be more susceptible to accumulate additional aberrations, which may enhance their ability to evolve into more malignant clones. As expected genomic arrays revealed unusually high

Table 9.2
Mutations and Outcome

N Mutations	CCyR (%)	MMR (%)	New Mutations (%)	FFS (%)
0/1	56	31	25	51
≥1	21	6	56	33

Abbreviations: N, number; CCyR, complete cytogenetic response; MMR, major molecular response; FFS, failure-free survival.

number of mutated genes in CML in blast crisis, but even CML in the chronic phase cells harbor numerous, yet sporadic aberrations (see Figs. 4.9 and 4.10). The latter observation strongly suggests that genomic instability in CML is an early event. TKI-resistant mutations in BCR–ABL1 kinase and additional chromosomal aberrations have been detected not only in LPCs, but also in LSCs suggesting that genomic instability occurs at the level of LSC and/or LPC.

Mutations detected in LSCs are likely to be passed on to successive generations of LPCs. Genomic instability usually results from enhanced DNA damage and/or deregulated mechanisms of DNA repair. Much endogenous DNA damage arises from reactive oxygen species (ROS), which can cause oxidative damage to all nucleobases and free nucleotides (such as 8-oxoG) generating mismatches and DNA double-strand breaks (DSBs). CD34+ CML cells display about three to eight times more oxidized nucleobases and four to eight times more DSBs than normal counterparts. Thus, elevation of ROS-induced oxidative DNA damage in CML cells appears to be a "driving force" of genomic instability.

Cellular DNA repair systems act to remove DNA damage and preserve the informational integrity of the genome. Since BCR–ABL1 kinase can suppress mismatch repair activity, elevated levels of oxidative DNA damage combined with inefficient mismatch repair activity may contribute to accumulation of point mutations in CML cells, including these in BCR–ABL1 kinase encoding TKI-resistant mutants. Oxidative DNA damage can also generate DSBs that

Table 9.3
Some of the Currently Established BCR–ABL1 Kinase Mutations

DNA Damaging Agents	DNA Lesions	Result	DNA Repair Mechanism
Alkylating agents	G-met	O6-methyl-G	MGMT
ROS/replication errors	T/C A/8-oxoguanine glycosylase	Mismatch Insertion Deletion	NMR
ROS/AID/X rays/ alkylating agent	8-oxoguanine glycosylase U	Oxidized base Uracil SSB	BER
ROS/UV light	T/T G/T	Bulky product (6-4) Photoproduct Intrastrand crosslink	NER
ROS/X rays/ cytostatics/ replication fork encountering a lesion	G/G	Interstrand crosslink DSB	HRR NHEJ SSA

Abbreviations: AID, activation-induced deaminase; BER, base excision repair; DSB, double strand break; HRR, homologous recombination repair; MGMT, 06-methylguanine-DNA methyltransferase; MMR, mismatch repair; NER, nucleotide excision repair; NHEJ, nonhomologous end joining; ROS, reactive oxygen species; SSA, single strand annealing.
Source: Data by courtesy of Professor Tomasz Skorski.

represent a "clear and present danger" to survival and genomic integrity. BCR–ABL1 kinase stimulates all three mechanisms of DSB repair: homologous recombination repair (HRR), nonhomologous end-joining (NHEJ) and single-strand annealing (SSA) to enhance genomic instability (Table 9.3). In leukemia cells HRR products incorporated point mutations, NHEJ resulted in more extensive deletions in some products and SSA generated large deletions. Thus, accelerated but unfaithful DSB repair may generate chromosomal aberrations, which are responsible for malignant progression of CML.

CONCLUSION

Resistance to TKIs therapy in patients with CML in chronic phase is uncommon, in contrast to those in the advanced phase of the disease. Primary resistance is very rare and most likely related either to the heterogeneity of the disease, or, as has been increasingly shown, due to poor compliance or adherence to the drug. In contrast, secondary or acquired resistance occurs much more frequently and often related to a mutation in BCR–ABL1 kinase domain.

The emergence of a mutation, particularly in patients who appear to be responding to imatinib, or indeed one of the second-generation TKIs, should not automatically be considered as a failure of treatment. Thus far Ph-positive subclones with over 80 different point mutations have been identified in leukemia cells obtained from patients with variable degrees of resistance to imatinib, and some of these, but by no means all, are clearly the cause of the resistance. Each mutation encodes a different amino acid substitution in the Abl kinase component of the BCR–ABL1 oncoprotein. Cells with the T315I mutation seem to be especially resistant to the inhibitory action of imatinib and all other currently available TKIs. Cells with other substitutions are relatively less resistant.

It is probable, but not confirmed, that some of these subclones pre-exist the administration of imatinib, or indeed any other TKI, but are allowed to expand when the unmutated oncoprotein molecule is inhibited by TKI; in other cases the mutation may develop *de novo* after initiation of TKI. There is also debate at present about the optimal treatment strategy for patients who remain in CCyR, on TKIs treatment, but develop a molecular relapse. It is likely that such a cohort may fare best either by increasing the dose of imatinib, or, as appears more likely, by switching to an alternative TKI. Studies in progress should help define this particular enigma in the near future.

Other potential topical preclinical challenges include the LSCs from patients with CML in chronic phase and/or LPCs, which may display elevated levels of ROS-induced oxidative DNA damage and inefficient/unfaithful DNA damage–repair mechanisms, which turn these cells into "ticking time-bombs," eventually producing TKI-resistant clones with an increased potential for progression to blast crisis.

In summary, imatinib has undoubtedly redefined the clinical management of patients with CML, but an increasing proportion of patients appear not to derive optimal benefit and a small minority do not respond to the drug at all. We have made some progress in elucidating the precise mechanisms of resistance in some patients, but clearly much more remains to be learned. Furthermore, we are now increasingly recognizing resistance with the second generation TKIs, the mechanisms of which might well be diverse. The ELN CML committee is currently preparing a document summarizing the definitions of response and resistance to the second-generation TKIs, which should be available by late 2013.

10 Concluding thoughts

For patients with *BCR–ABL1*-positive leukemias, which comprise all the Ph chromosome-positive and some Ph-negative leukemias, the introduction of the original tyrosine kinase inhibitor (TKI), imatinib, into the clinics in 1998, resulted in being both a classic and a landmark achievement. It was classic since it established the notion of the BCR–ABL1 being of a principal pathogenetic importance, and a landmark, since it established the usefulness of TKIs to accord a survival benefit to the majority of patients with chronic myeloid leukemia (CML) in chronic phase. This is even more remarkable, given the considerable skepticism expressed, from both academic and industry experts, about any possible clinical value of TKIs in the early 1990s!

After 12 months of therapy with imatinib, 69% of patients with CML in chronic phase achieve a complete cytogenetic response (CCyR), and after eight years of follow-up, such response rates increase to 83%. This remarkable activity translates into an estimated overall survival of 93% (when only CML-related deaths are accounted for), which is substantially higher than that achieved by any previous medical treatment, including allogeneic stem cell transplant (SCT). The success in the treatment of patients with CML in advanced phases and the Ph-positive acute lymphoblastic leukemia (ALL) has also been improved with the addition of imatinib to cytotoxic drugs, although less remarkably.

The adverse events attributable to imatinib, and indeed dasatinib and nilotinib (so far), appear to be relatively mild, but not innocuous, and generally easily manageable. In contrast, intolerance and resistance, in particular secondary, have been more challenging, with about a third of all patients with CML in chronic phase and substantially higher proportions with CML in advanced phases and Ph-positive ALL, not being able to tolerate imatinib or have a leukemia that becomes resistant or refractory to imatinib; precise data on the use of second-generation TKI are currently not known, but probably better compared with imatinib, albeit with a relatively short period of follow-up.

Current observations suggest that about 20% of imatinib-treated patients never achieve a CCyR, and 10% who do will lose such a response over time. Furthermore, about 26% of patients are intolerant to imatinib. Novel risk stratification methods and optimal molecular monitoring can be used to judge response and predict future risk of progression for patients with CML in chronic phase. These are complemented by recent insights into the mechanisms of resistance to TKIs as well as by knowledge gained regarding aspects of the cellular and molecular biology of BCR–ABL1-positive cells, such as their underlying genomic instability. Given the limited activity of TKI therapy in advanced phases of the disease, the most immediate goal of CML therapy is the prevention of progression, which has been associated with the achievement of deep responses at early time points during the course of TKI therapy. In this regard, the use of second-generation TKIs as first-line therapy has led to an increase in the number of patients capable of achieving a complete molecular response (CMR). It is likely, though not confirmed, that some of these patients, who have been in CMR for about 2 years, might be potential candidates for discontinuing TKI therapy. A current study demonstrate that over half of CML patients in CMR on imatinib relapse quickly when TKI therapy is stopped. It is postulated, but not proved, that these relapses are a consequence of quiescent CML stem cells that are resistant to killing by conventional TKIs. Indeed, these malignant progenitors can be detected in the bone marrow from CML patients in CCyR on imatinib.

Studies have demonstrated the presence of BCR–ABL1-positive clonogenic progenitors, including LTCIC in CML patients in CMR, whose disease is undetectable by conventional polymerase chain reaction (PCR) technology. Hence, there is much interest in identifying targets and strategies for eliminating leukemic stem cells (LSCs) in CML. Several groups have reported on using next-generation and deep sequencing technologies to interrogate CML patient genomes to identify new pathogenetic targets in CML. Comparative whole transcriptome sequencing of a CML patient who progressed to myeloid blast crisis identified eight mis-sense mutations in novel genes, including *IDH2* and protein kinase D2. Deep sequencing of 40 blast crisis CML patients (25 myeloid, 10 lymphoid, 5 unspecified) revealed frequent *IKZF1*, *RUNX1*, and *ASXL1* mutations that developed during disease progression. Further studies will be necessary to determine the role of these mutations in disease progression and assess their suitability as targets for therapy.

Additional research efforts have focused on specific signaling pathways that might be targets for elimination of LSCs in CML. For example, BCL6, a zinc finger protein that functions as a proto-oncogene in diffuse large B-cell lymphoma, has been shown to be required for maintenance of CML stem cells in a retroviral mouse model, and incubation of human CML progenitors with a peptide BCL6 inhibitor decreased engraftment of immunodeficient NSG mice. Stearoyl-CoA desaturase 1 (Scd1), an endoplasmic reticulum enzyme catalyzing the biosynthesis of monounsaturated fatty acids from saturated fatty acids, was identified as a potential tumor suppressor gene in CML stem cells, as CML-like leukemia induced by *Scd1–/–* BM had higher levels of functional LSCs, whereas treatment of leukemic mice with the PPARγ agonist rosiglitazone increased Scd1 expression and decreased LSCs. Several previous studies have implicated the Hedgehog (Hh) pathway in the maintenance of CML stem cells in mouse retroviral models.

The phenotype of leukemia-initiating cells in a conditional transgenic mouse model of CML has been recently defined and demonstrated that treatment of mice with the Hh inhibitor LDE225 together with nilotinib decreased phenotypic CML LSCs in spleen, but not bone marrow, and further decreased engraftment of NSG mice with human CD34+ CML progenitors. Given the recent launch of clinical trials of Hh pathway antagonists in refractory Ph-positive leukemia, further preclinical studies of these agents are warranted to aid in their clinical development. The possible role of JAK2 in the maintenance of quiescent, TKI-resistant BCR–ABL1-expressing stem cells in CML was also explored by several groups, where JAK2 may be activated by an extrinsic pathway through stroma-mediated

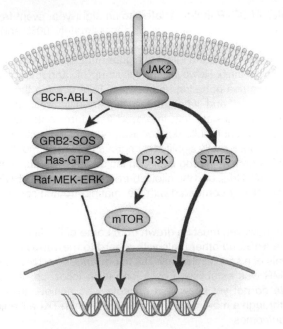

Figure 10.1
Schematic representation of STAT5 activation in Ph-positive chronic myeloid leukemia: BCR–ABL1 phosphorylates STAT5 at the same critical tyrosine residue close to the SH2 domain, inducing the same downstream events independently of JAK2.
Source: *Courtesy of Dr Doriano Fabbro. A color version of this figure can be found in* Plate VIII *between pages 46 and 47.*

cytokines or through an intrinsic pathway via inhibition of a protein phosphatase, PP2A. These results open the possibility of targeting JAK2 in CML either through a specific JAK2 TKI or through the PP2A activator FTY720. Indeed, there are now several clinical trials assessing the combinations of BCR–ABL1 TKIs and JAK inhibitors, such as ruxolitinib (Fig. 10.1). Together, these exciting basic and preclinical studies continue to define CML as, perhaps, the best understood human cancer and offer the hope that one day we might be able to eradicate the leukemia and "cure" patients without the need for lifelong drug therapy.

The natural history of all BCR–ABL1-positive leukemias has been modified positively by the introduction of TKI therapy, which renders high rates of CCyR that translate into an eight-year event-free survival and overall survival rates of approximately 80% and 85%, respectively. Second-generation TKIs, such as dasatinib and nilotinib, produce CCyR and MMR at higher rates and at a much faster pace than imatinib. However, the follow-up of randomized studies involving the use of second-generation TKIs used in the first-line setting is short and whether the higher initial response rates observed will translate into improved long-term outcomes is yet unknown. Current results do, however, demonstrate either a trend toward or a statistically significant improvement at 12 months in the rates of freedom from progression in the dasatinib-treated cohort in the DASISION trial, and the nilotinib-treated cohort in the ENESTnd trail, respectively, compared with the imatinib-treated cohorts.

Caution, however, must be drawn from some of the lessons learnt from the IRIS and other trials with regard to the various timelines and goals of a specific therapy. The importance of achieving CCyR and MMR was established by a long-term follow-up of the IRIS trial. We do not yet know that patients who achieve these endpoints through a more potent second-generation TKI will enjoy the same outcomes.

It is perhaps somewhat daunting that the current wave of second-generation TKI trials differs in study designs, how the results are censored and perhaps, more importantly, the selection of different primary endpoints (e.g., MMR in ENESTnd and "confirmed" CCyR in DASISION), which are evaluated at specific time points. The longer-term impact of MMR, in contrast to CCyR, is unknown at present, although it may turn out to be more robust in terms of predicting survival.

Efforts are addressing potential strategies to eradicate the quiescent CML stem cells, which appear to be resistant to all currently available TKIs. These include combining TKIs with other agents, old and new, for patients with CML in chronic phase, in addition to consider various ways in which TKIs could be combined or used in sequence. It is of some interest that in addition to assessing combinations with novel agents such as histone deacetylase inhibitors, antagonists of the hedgehog signaling pathway, inhibitors of autophagy, JAK2 inhibitors, considerable efforts are evaluating interferon-α (IFN-α), both as part of initial therapy and also once a CMR has been achieved.

The French SPIRIT trial assessed the potential to combine IFN-α with TKI as initial first-line therapy. Interim analysis of this trial has demonstrated statistically significant improvements in MMR and CMR rates for the combination treatment compared with imatinib 400 mg daily. It is of note that although these results have been confirmed by the Italian GIMEMA group, the German CML IV trial did not find any benefit in combining IFN-α to imatinib 400 mg daily.

As our efforts in improving on the primary therapies continue, we can anticipate an improvement in the way progression and resistance to TKI risk are classified, based on the emerging tools. These tools may include of set of different levels of genetics-mutated genes that become evident in studies utilizing whole genome sequencing, microRNAs, and gene expression. In addition, the advent of DNA sequencing may uncover new cryptic translocations, or splicing variants, which define disease biology.

Molecular monitoring by RT-qPCR is now widely adopted as a monitoring tool and in many parts of the world supplanting conventional cytogenetics. In the future, cytogenetics will probably still be useful to define new clonal abnormalities associated with advanced-phase disease, until, perhaps, the whole genome sequencing becomes a relatively rapid and cost-effective tool. PCR is now routinely carried out on peripheral blood samples.

Recent studies, such as the French group's Stop Imatinib (STIM) and the ELN's European Stop Tyrosine Kinase Inhibitors (EURO-SKI) trials, suggest that achieving a CMR may predict for greater durability of response and perhaps be used to interrupt TKI therapy. Clearly, this is of paramount importance since it could allow patients to discontinue TKI therapy safely once a CMR has been achieved. The updated results of STIM study in December 2012 suggest that in about 40% of patients who achieve a CMR, imatinib could be discontinued safely (Fig. 5.5). Conversely, about

60% of patients relapse at a molecular level within six months of imatinib being discontinued. This makes CMR an attractive target for both clinicians and patients. Efforts to develop more sensitive molecular methods, on RNA (disease specific) or DNA (patient specific), to better assess the depths of CMR are in progress. It is tempting to speculate that such a strategy may represent a "cure" for patients with CML in chronic phase.

Bibliography

Al-Kali A, Kantarjian H, Shan J, et al. Current event-free survival after sequential tyrosine kinase inhibitor therapy for chronic myeloid leukemia. Cancer 2011; 117: 327–35.

Apperley JF. Part I: mechanisms of resistance to imatinib in chronic myeloid leukaemia. Lancet Oncol 2007; 8: 1018–29.

Baccarani M, Cortes J, Pane F, et al. Chronic myeloid leukemia: an update of concepts and management recommendations of European LeukemiaNet. J Clin Oncol 2009; 27: 6041–51.

Cortes J, Hochaus A, Hughes T, Kantarjian H. Front-line and salvage therapies with tyrosine kinase inhibitors and other treatments in chronic myeloid leukemia. J Clin Oncol 2011; 29: 524–31.

Druker BJ, Guilhot F, O'Brien SG, et al. Five-year follow-up of patients receiving imatinib for chronic myeloid leukemia. N Engl J Med 2006; 355: 2408–17.

Druker BJ, Talpaz M, Resta DJ, et al. Efficacy and safety of a specific inhibitor of the BCR-ABL tyrosine kinase in chronic myeloid leukemia. N Engl J Med 2001; 344: 1031–7.

Fabarius A, Leitner A, Hochhaus A, et al. Schweizerische Arbeitsgemeinschaft für Klinische Krebsforschung (SAKK) and the German CML Study Group. Impact of additional cytogenetic aberrations at diagnosis on prognosis of CML: long-term observation of 1151 patients from the randomized CML Study IV. Blood 2011; 118: 6760–8; Epub 2011 Oct 28.

Goldman JM, Mughal TI. Chronic myeloid leukaemia. In: Hoffbrand AV, Catovsky D, Tuddenham EGD, Green AR, eds. Postgraduate Haematology 6E. Wiley, Chichester, 2010: 483–502.

Goldman JM. Ponatinib for Chronic Myeloid Leukemia. N Engl J Med 2012; 367: 2148–9.

Gratwohl A, Hermans J, Goldman JM, et al. Risk assessment for patients with chronic myeloid leukaemia before allogeneic blood or marrow transplantation. Chronic leukemia working party of the European

Group for Blood and Marrow Transplantation. Lancet 1998; 352: 1087–92.

Hasford J, Pfirrmann M, Hehlmann R, et al. A new prognostic score for survival of patients with chronic myeloid leukemia treated with interferon alfa. Writing Committee for the Collaborative CML Prognostic Factors Project Group. J Natl Cancer Inst 1998; 90: 850–8.

Hasford J, Baccarani M, Hoffmann V, et al. Predicting complete cytogenetic response and subsequent progression-free survival in 2060 patients with CML on imatinib treatment: the EUTOS score. Blood 2011; 118: 686–92.

Hehlmann R. CML in the imatinib era. Best Pract Res Clin Hematol 2009; 22: 283–4.

Hochhaus A, Saglio G, le Coutre P, et al. Superior efficacy of nilotinib compared with imatinib in newly diagnosed patients with chronic myeloid leukemia in chronic (CML-CP); ENESTnd minimum 24-month follow-up. Haematologica 2011; 96: 203–4.

Horn M, Glauche I, Muller MC, et al. Model-based decision rules reduces the risk of molecular relapse after cessation of tyrosine kinase inhibitor therapy in chronic myeloid leukemia. Blood 2013; 121: 378–84.

Jabbour E, Cortes J, Santos FP, et al. Results of allogeneic hematopoietic stem cell transplantation for chronic myelogenous leukemia patients who failed tyrosine kinase inhibitors after developing BCR-ABL1 kinase domain mutations. Blood 2011; 117: 3641–7.

Jabbour E, Cortes J, Nazha A, et al. EUTOS score is not predictive for survival and outcome in patients with early chronic phase chronic myeloid leukemia treated with tyrosine kinase inhibitors: a single institution experience. Blood 2012; 119: 4524–6.

Jelinek J, Gharibyan V, Estecio MR, et al. Aberrant DNA methylation is associated with disease progression, resistance to imatinib and shortened survival in chronic myelogenous leukemia. PLoS One 2011; 6: e22110; Epub 2011 Jul 8.

Kantarjian H, Baccarani M, Jabbour E, Saglio G, Cortes J. Second-generation Tyrsoine Kinase inhibitors: the future of frontline CML therapy. Clin Cancer Res 2011; 17: 1674–83.

Kantarjian H, O'Brien S, Jabbour E, et al. Improved survival in chronic myeloid leukemia since the introduction of imatinib therapy: a single institution historical experience. Blood 2012; 119: 1981–7.

Kantarjian H, Shah NP, Hochhaus A, et al. Dasatinib versus imatinib in newly diagnosed chronic-phase chronic myeloid leukemia. N Engl J Med 2010; 362: 2260–70.

Kantarjian HM, O'Brien S, Cortes JE, et al. Complete cytogenetic and molecular responses to interferon-alpha-based therapy for chronic myelogenous leukemia are associated with excellent long-term prognosis. Cancer 2003; 97: 1033–41.

Kantarjian HM, Shah NP, Cortes JE, et al. Dasatinib or imatinib in newly diagnosed chronic-phase chronic myeloid leukemia: 2-year follow-up from a randomized phase 3 trial (DASISION). Blood 2012; 119: 1123–9.

Krause DS, Van Etten RA. Bedside to bench: interfering with leukemic stem cells. Nat Med 2008; 14: 494–5.

Mahon FX, Réa D, Guilhot J, et al. Intergroupe Français des Leucémies Myéloïdes Chroniques. Discontinuation of imatinib in patients with chronic myeloid leukaemia who have maintained complete molecular remission for at least 2 years: the prospective, multicentre Stop Imatinib (STIM) trial. Lancet Oncol 2010; 11: 1029–35; Epub 2010 Oct 19.

Mahon FX, Réa D, Guilhot J, et al. Discontinuation of imatinib in patients with chronic myeloid leukaemia who have maintained complete molecular remission for at least 2 years: the prospective, multicentre Stop Imatinib (STIM) trial. Lancet Oncol 2010; 11: 1029–35.

Marin D, Bazeos A, Mahon FX, et al. Adherence is the critical factor for achieving molecular responses in patients with chronic myeloid leukemia who achieve complete cytogenetic responses on imatinib. J Clin Oncol 2010; 28: 2381–8.

Marin D, Ibrahim A, Lucas C, et al. Assessment of BCR-ABL1 transcript levels at 3 months is the only requirement for predicting outcome for patients with chronic myeloid leukemia treated with tyrosine kinase inhibitors. J Clin Oncol 2011; 30: 232–8.

Milojkovic D, Nicholson E, Apperley JF, et al. Early prediction of success or failure of treatment with second-generation tyrosine kinase inhibitors in patients with chronic myeloid leukemia. Haematologica 2010; 95: 224–31.

Mughal TI, Yong A, Szydlo R, et al. RT-PCR studies in patients with chronic myeloid leukemia in remission 5 years after allogeneic stem cell transplant define risk of subsequent relapse. Br J Haematol 200l; 115: 569–74.

Mughal TI, Radich JP, Van Etten RA, et al. Successes, challenges, and strategies – proceedings of the 5th Annual BCR-ABL1 positive and BCR-ABL negative myeloproliferative neoplasms workshop. Am J Hematol 2011; 86: 811–6.

Mughal TI, Schreiber A. Long term toxicity of imatinib when used as a first line therapy myeloid leukemia. Biologics 2010; 4: 315–23.

Mughal TI, Goldman JM. Chronic Myeloid Leukaemia in Oxford Textbook of Medicine Ed. Warrell, Cox & Firth, Oxford University Press, 6th Edition, 2013.

Nicolini FE, Mauro MJ, Martinelli G, et al. Epidemiologic study on survival of chronic myeloid leukemia and Ph(+) acute lymphoblastic leukemia patients with BCR-ABL T315I mutation. Blood 2009; 114: 5271–8.

Nowell PC, Hungerford DA. Chromosome studies on normal and leukemic human leukocytes. J Natl Cancer Inst 1960; 25: 85–109.

O'Brien S, Abboud CN, Berman E, et al. Chronic myelogenous leukemia. National Comprehensive Cancer Network. 2010. [Available from: http://www.nccn.org/professionals/physician_gls/f_guidelines.asp]

O'Brien SG, Guilhot F, Larson RA, et al. Imatinib compared with interferon and low-dose cytarabine for newly diagnosed chronic-phase myeloid leukemia. N Engl J Med 2003; 348: 994–1004.

Okimoto RA, Van Etten RA. Navigating the road toward optimal initial therapy for chronic myeloid leukemia. Curr Opin Hematol 2011; 18: 89–97.

Pavlů J, Szydlo R, Goldman JM, et al. Three decades of transplantation for chronic myeloid leukemia: what have we learned? Blood 2011; 117: 755–63.

Perrotti D, Jamieson C, Goldman J, Skorski T. Chronic myeloid leukemia: mechanisms of blastic transformation. J Clin Invest 2010; 120: 2254–64.

Quintás-Cardama A, Jabbour EJ. Considerations for early switch to nilotinib or dasatinib in patients with chronic myeloid leukemia with inadequate response to first-line imatinib. Leuk Res 2013; pre-published on line 6 February 2013.

Saglio G, Kim DW, Issaragrisil S, et al. Nilotinib versus imatinib for newly diagnosed chronic myeloid leukemia. N Engl J Med 2010; 362: 2251–9.

Savage D, Szydlo R, Goldman JM, et al. Clinical features at diagnosis of 430 patients with chronic myeloid leukemia seen at a referral centre over a 16-year period. Br J Haematol 1997; 96: 111–16.

Shah NP, Tran C, Lee FY, et al. Overriding imatinib resistance with a novel ABL kinase inhibitor. Science 2004; 305: 399–401.

Soverini S, Hochhaus A, Nicolini F, et al. BCR-ABL kinase domain mutation analysis in chronic myeloid leukemia patients treated with tyrosine kinase inhibitors: recommendations from an expert panel on behalf of European LeukemiaNet. Blood 2011; 118: 1208–15.

Sokal JE, Cox EB, Baccarani M, et al. Prognostic discrimination in 'good-risk' chronic granulocytic leukemia. Blood 1984; 63: 789–99.

Stein AM, Bottino D, Modur V, et al. BCR-ABL transcript dynamics support the hypothesis that leukemic stem cells are reduced during imatinib treatment. Clin Cancer Res 2011; 17: 6812–21.

Yong AS, Szydlo RM, Goldman JM, Apperley JF, Melo JV. Molecular profiling of CD34+ cells identifies low expression of CD7, along with high expression of proteinase 3 or elastase, as predictors of longer survival in patients with CML. Blood 2006; 107: 205–12.

Index